the

GESTATIONAL DIABETES

Cookbook & Meal Plan

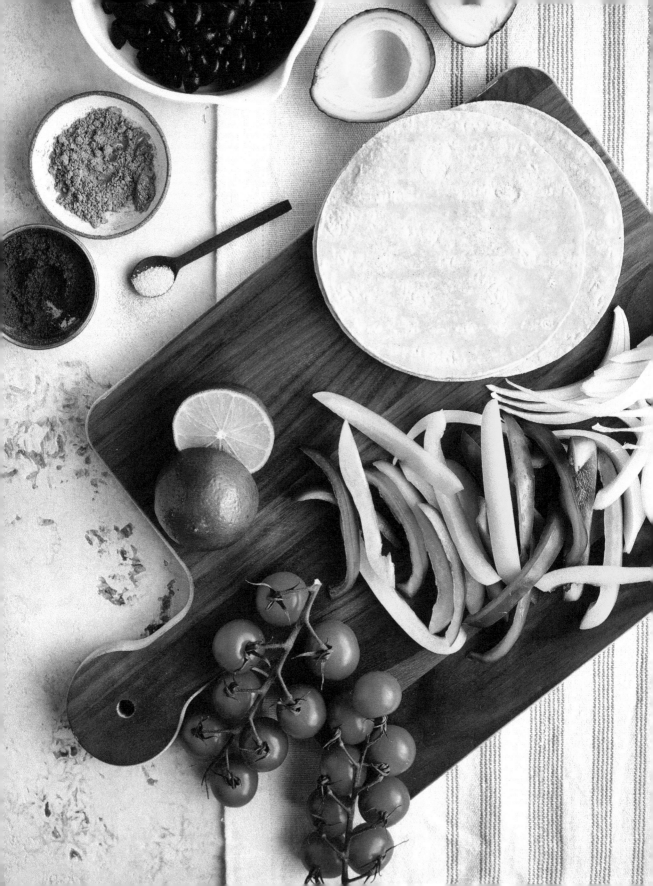

the
GESTATIONAL DIABETES
Cookbook & Meal Plan

A BALANCED EATING GUIDE FOR YOU AND YOUR BABY

by Joanna Foley, RD, and Traci Houston

PHOTOGRAPHY BY HELENE DUJARDIN

ROCKRIDGE PRESS

Interior and Cover Designer: Amanda Kirk
Photo Art Director/Art Manager: Michael Hardgrove
Editor: Eliza Kirby
Production Editor: Edgar Doolan
Photography: Helene Dujardin
Food Styling: Anna Hampton

ISBN: Print 978-1-64152-494-0
eBook 978-1-64152-495-7

To my amazing daughter, Maiyanni.
The experience and this opportunity
never would have come without you.
You are my inspiration!

—TRACI HOUSTON

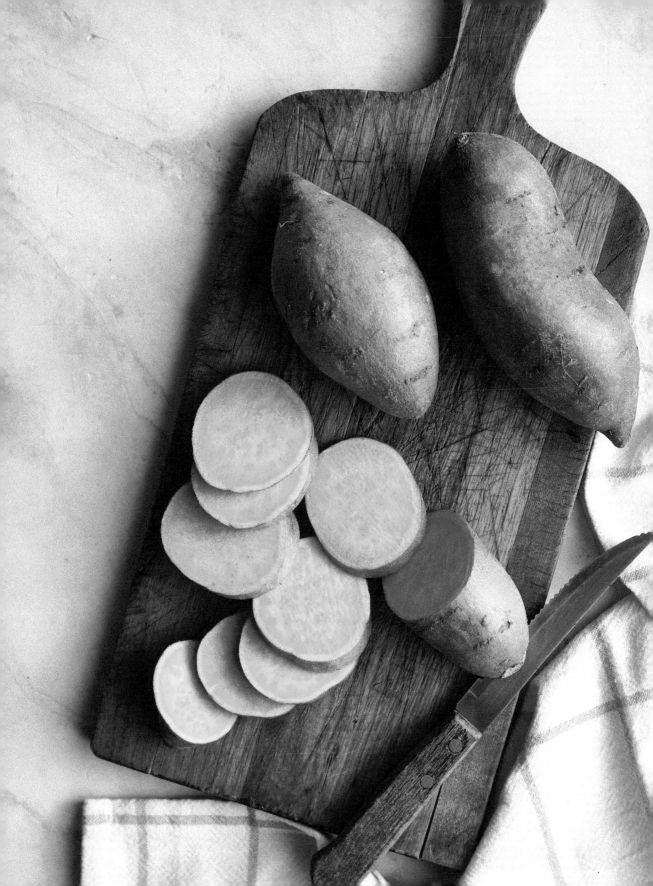

Contents

Introduction

You Have Control

A diagnosis of gestational diabetes can be scary. Believe me; I know.

My name is Traci Houston. I was about 24 weeks into my first pregnancy when I was diagnosed with gestational diabetes mellitus (GDM). I had never heard of GDM, but my doctor said my test results were "off the charts."

I left my doctor's office feeling uninformed, confused, and worried. My doctor had given me a referral to a dietitian, but it would be weeks before the dietitian could see me. In the meantime, I was desperate for practical advice about how to manage the diagnosis.

Unfortunately, my story is not uncommon. Sometimes it's hard to get the care we need when we need it. And, of course, we all have busy, stressful lives. As I struggled to find useful information, I was also finishing culinary school, planning for my baby, and feeling utterly exhausted. I felt—perhaps as you do—that the last thing I needed was another boulder to carry.

After the birth of my daughter, I wanted to prevent other women with GDM from suffering from a lack of resources. That desire drove me to start a recipe blog for women with gestational diabetes. It is also the impetus behind this book.

Here's the thing: You can't control whether you have gestational diabetes, but you *can* control how you manage the diagnosis, and you *can* have a healthy pregnancy.

What to Expect and How This Book Can Help

Having gestational diabetes means you have to adjust your relationship with food and your eating habits. It may sound overwhelming, but don't worry. In the following chapters, my coauthor, Joanna Foley, a registered dietitian, clearly explains the nutritional concepts you need to understand to navigate your diagnosis. The meal plan, helpful charts, shopping lists, and recipes are developed to support your dietary requirements and make the transition easy.

The meal plan also keeps you on track so you can focus your attention on the rest of your busy life. Nutrition facts, substitutions, and tips will help you establish habits that will carry you through the rest of your pregnancy and beyond.

Although diet is the central concern of this book, be sure to remember exercise. Exercise assists in regulating your blood sugar. Consult your health care team about what is right for you.

The goal of this book is to empower you to effectively manage this diagnosis through a whole-food diet and deliver a healthy baby.

So take a deep breath, stay positive, and enjoy this time. You got this.

ASK THE REGISTERED DIETITIAN: WHAT IS GDM AND WHAT ARE ITS RISKS?

Gestational diabetes mellitus (GDM) is a disorder of blood sugar regulation that occurs during pregnancy for some women. According to a 2014 analysis by the Centers for Disease Control and Prevention, it is estimated to occur in about 9 percent of pregnant women. It is generally diagnosed around the 24th week of gestation and occurs as a result of the body not being able to make and use the amount of insulin it needs during pregnancy. If left untreated or poorly controlled, gestational diabetes can lead to health risks for both mother and baby, including preterm birth, high birth weight, and other birth complications. In addition, women with gestational diabetes and their children are more likely to develop type 2 diabetes later in life. Treatment options involve diet and lifestyle modifications as well as medications, including insulin, if needed.

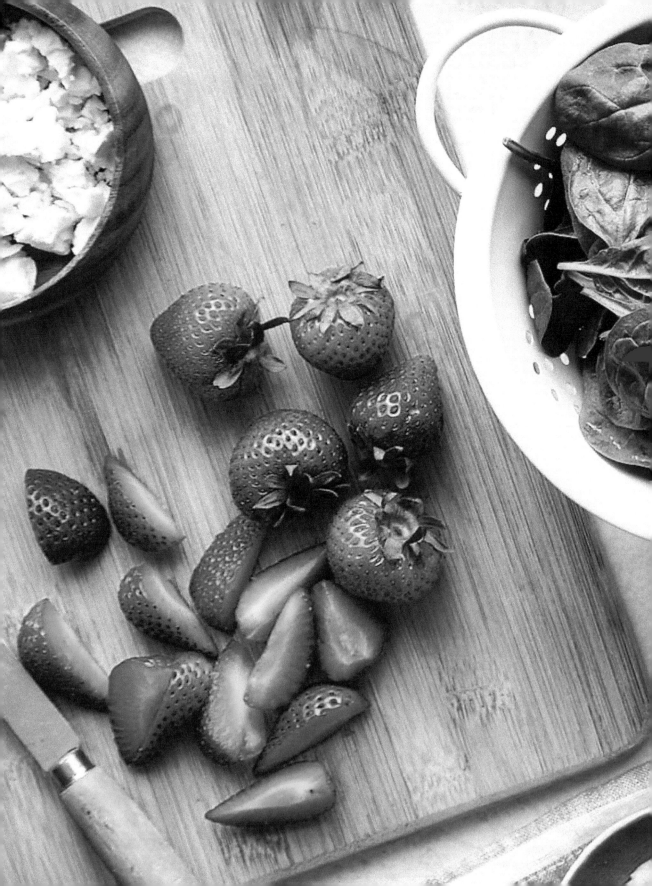

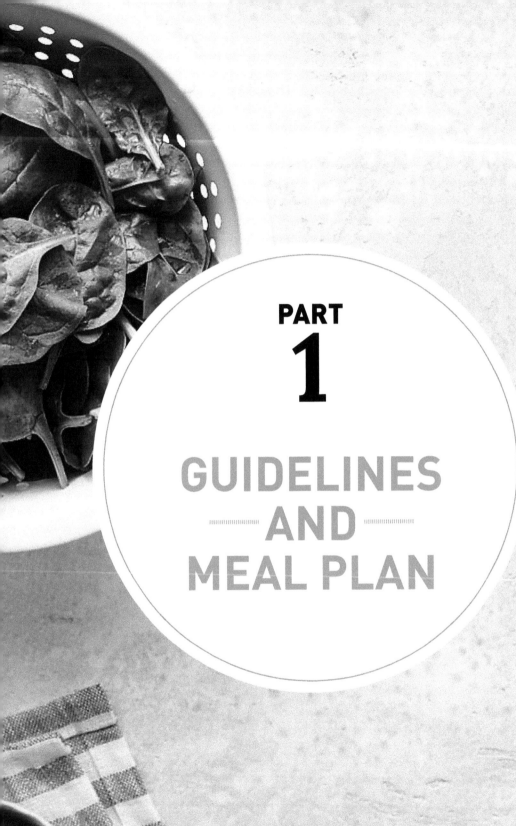

PART
1

GUIDELINES
AND
MEAL PLAN

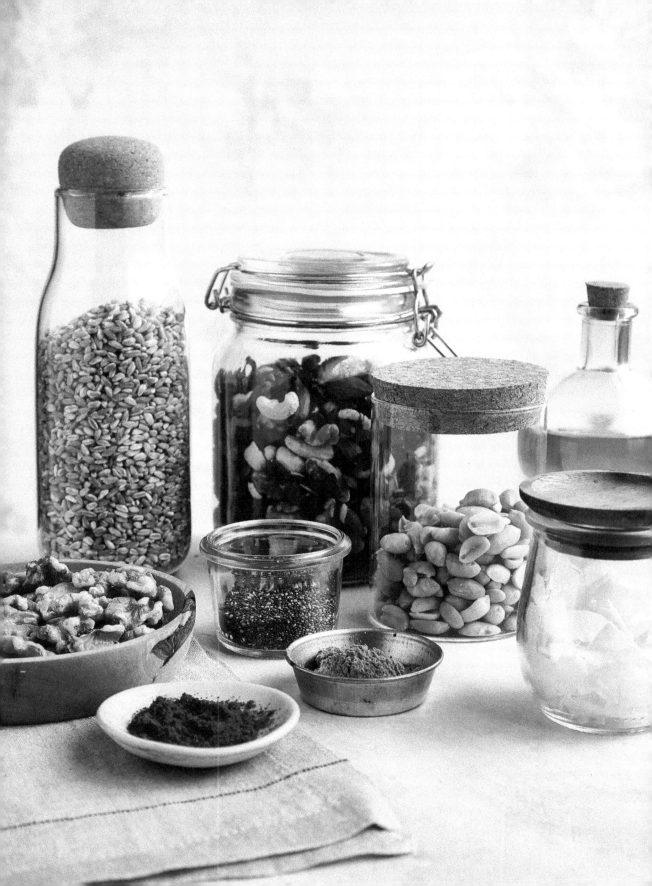

CHAPTER ONE

Eating Guidelines for Gestational Diabetes

As a registered dietitian, I've worked with many patients with gestational diabetes, so I know this diagnosis can be overwhelming. You might be worried you will have to go on insulin or follow an especially restrictive diet. You may be anxious about your baby's health. If you've had any of these feelings, I am here to tell you that you are not alone and that there is hope. This book will provide you with the tools you need to jumpstart your health journey, rid you of your fears, and manage your diagnosis using the best medicine of all—your diet.

A diagnosis of gestational diabetes is both temporary and manageable through diet and lifestyle changes. Your doctor will work with you to ensure you're on the right track, but you can also take meaningful action on your own. You *can* have gestational diabetes and give birth to a healthy baby by making smart food choices and managing your blood sugar—and you can eat delicious food at the same time.

The concepts and meals provided in this book are based on a "real-food" approach. Conventional diabetic diets often consist of "sugar-free" products made with harmful artificial sweeteners. They also place emphasis on carbohydrate count alone, without focusing on the quality or proper combinations of foods consumed. The real-food approach emphasizes natural and minimally processed ingredients and focuses on quality of carbohydrates consumed, not just quantity. As you will learn, 30 grams of carbohydrates from a sugar-laden pastry does not impact the body the same way as 30 grams of carbohydrates from brown rice and a vegetable stir-fry. Additionally, this approach promotes a balance of protein, carbohydrates, and fat as essential to managing blood sugar and takes the emphasis off of just carbohydrates alone. Most importantly, this book takes the focus off of restriction and teaches you how to enjoy foods that you love in a nourishing and satisfying way.

The following guidelines will give you the information necessary to establish and maintain healthy everyday eating habits. You'll learn about carb control, the basics of creating a balanced meal, and foods to enjoy or limit for blood sugar management. Practical information and plenty of helpful tips will help take the guesswork out of what to eat from day to day and from meal to meal, so you can focus your energy on your pregnancy. Are you excited yet? You should be!

Carb Control

Managing gestational diabetes isn't only about carbs, but it is important to recognize that out of the three macronutrients—carbohydrates, protein, and fat—*only carbohydrates will raise your blood sugar.* It's important to consider the amount of carbs in each snack and meal you eat. To effectively control your carbohydrate intake, you first need to learn the difference between complex and simple carbohydrates. You will also need to understand how many grams of carbs you can have each day, how to distribute carbs across meals, and when to check your blood sugar.

Carbohydrates come in different forms, and some are healthier than others. Starches and fiber, or "complex carbohydrates," are better for you because they have a low glycemic index, meaning they cause a slower rise in blood sugar. Sugars, on the other hand, or "simple carbohydrates," have a high glycemic index and tend to raise blood sugar levels quickly. It is best to stick to complex carbohydrates as much as possible.

COMPLEX CARBOHYDRATES

- » Fruit (whole and in its natural form)
- » Legumes (such as beans, lentils, and peanuts)
- » Nonstarchy vegetables (such as bell peppers, Brussels sprouts, and spinach)
- » Nuts
- » Starchy vegetables (such as corn, peas, and sweet potatoes)
- » Whole grains

SIMPLE CARBOHYDRATES

- » Added sugar (of all kinds)
- » Desserts
- » Pastries
- » Refined grains (such as white flour)
- » Sugary beverages (such as juice and soda)

One serving of carbohydrates is equal to 15 grams. Our meal plan adheres to the following general guidelines:

- » Breakfast, 30 grams (2 servings)
- » Lunch, 30 to 45 grams (2 to 3 servings)
- » Dinner, 30 to 45 grams (2 to 3 servings)
- » Snack, 10 to 15 grams (1 serving)

Your total daily carbs should not exceed about 150 grams, an amount that has been shown to be effective at managing blood sugar while also meeting your essential nutrient requirements during pregnancy. However, your individual needs may be slightly different depending on your age, body size, activity level, and weeks of gestation. Working with a registered dietitian can help you determine what's best for you.

The best way to know how many carbohydrates you need is to check your blood sugar. I recommend checking shortly after waking up and before eating, then again about two hours after a meal. If your readings are low, you may need slightly more carbohydrates. If your blood sugar is running high, you will need to reduce your carbohydrate intake by adjusting the type and amount of carbs being consumed. Your doctor will explain what normal readings should be throughout the day.

The good news? Modifying your carb intake can be simple, and it doesn't require any special equipment.

READING NUTRITION LABELS

Understanding nutrition labels is essential to managing your blood sugar and health during pregnancy. Here's what to look for:

1. **Serving size:** If the serving size is ½ cup and you usually eat closer to 1 cup, make sure to double the amount of carbs and other nutrients listed.

2. **Calories per serving:** Compare calories to choose the best option for you.

3. **Total carbohydrate:** This number includes all forms of carbohydrates: dietary fiber, total sugars, and added sugars. Because all types of carbohydrates affect blood sugar levels, use total grams when determining portion size. **Dietary fiber** can help balance and improve blood sugar response. At least 28 grams per day are recommended during pregnancy. Limiting **total sugar** as much as possible will have the largest impact on your blood sugar levels. Limit **added sugars** the most; they are less beneficial than naturally occurring sugars. The American Heart Association recommends women consume no more than 25 grams or 6 teaspoons per day, but the less, the better.

4. **Protein:** Balancing carbohydrates with protein can help stabilize blood sugar.

5. **Fat:** Choose products that contain mostly unsaturated fat. Limit saturated fat from animal products and avoid trans fat.

6. **Sodium:** GDM increases your risk of developing high blood pressure and pre-eclampsia. Sodium is also closely linked to an increased risk of these conditions. Pay close attention and make a concerted effort to consume less than 2,300 milligrams or 1 teaspoon per day.

Nutrition Facts

20 servings per container

Serving size   2/3 Cup (90g)

Amount per serving

Calories   80

	% Daily Value*
Total Fat 2.5g	3%
Saturated Fat 0g	0%
Trans Fat 0g	
Cholesterol 0mg	0%
Sodium 15mg	1%
Total Carbohydrate 10g	4%
Dietary Fiber 5g	18%
Total Sugars 3g	
Includes 0g Added Sugars	0%
Protein 5g	
Vitamin D 0mcg	0%
Calcium 30mg	2%
Iron 1mg	6%
Potassium 280mg	6%

*The % Daily Value tells you how much a nutrient in a serving of food contributes to a daily diet. 2000 calories a day is used for general nutrition advice.

Calories per gram:
Fat 9 • Carbohydrate 4 • Protein 4

What Is a Balanced Meal?

By now you understand the role carbohydrates play in your blood sugar levels, but they aren't the whole picture.

Managing blood sugar is a unique balance between choosing the best sources of carbohydrates and strategically pairing them with the right sources of protein and fat. Healthy protein and fat help lower the blood sugar response and promote satiety, or a feeling of fullness, which prevents overeating. Proteins and fats also contain different nutrients than carbohydrates, so preparing meals that balance proteins and fats with carbohydrates will help you manage your blood sugar and give you the biggest nutritional "bang for your buck."

Protein exists in animal and plant-based sources, and both are important during pregnancy. Plant-based protein sources also contain fiber, which is beneficial for managing blood sugar levels. Animal proteins are also extremely nutritious and provide all of the essential amino acids you and your baby need. When it comes to fat, unsaturated is best. Saturated fat, while not as healthy as unsaturated fat, can still be consumed safely in moderation. Trans fat, however, offers no nutritional benefit and should be avoided completely. Be on the lookout for any ingredients that include the words *hydrogenated* and *partially hydrogenated*, and try to stay away from them.

You have probably heard about common foods to avoid during pregnancy. Having gestational diabetes is no exception to those recommendations. Furthermore, a diet high in fat or sodium will not promote optimal health, weight, or blood sugar control, regardless of how few carbohydrates you eat. So it's a good idea to avoid highly processed or fried foods and most fast food.

For specific examples of foods that fit these categories, see "Foods That Are Good for You and Your Baby" (page 8), "Foods to Eat in Moderation" (page 9), and "Foods to Avoid" (page 10).

CARBS* (PROVIDES ~15 GRAMS OF CARBS/SERVING)	PROTEINS	FATS	BEVERAGES
Berries (1 cup)†	Beans or lentils (½ cup)	Avocado (½)	Almond milk, unsweetened (1 cup)
Fruit (whole), such as apples, pears, oranges, kiwis, or peaches (1 small)	Cheese (1 ounce)	Chia seeds or flaxseed (1 to 2 tablespoons)	Decaf coffee (8 ounces)
Leafy greens or other nonstarchy vegetables (unlimited)	Chicken breast (4 ounces)	Coconut milk (½ cup)	Decaf tea (unlimited)
Oats (½ cup cooked)	Edamame, shelled (½ cup)	Coconut, shredded (¼ cup)	
Starchy vegetables, such as sweet potato, corn, or peas (½ cup)	Greek yogurt (6 ounces)	Nut butter (2 tablespoons)	Water, including sparkling and unsweetened flavored water (unlimited)
Whole grains, such as quinoa, whole-wheat pasta, or brown rice (⅓ cup cooked)	Lean all-natural beef or pork (4 ounces)	Nuts or seeds (1 ounce or ¼ cup)	
Whole-grain English muffin or pita bread (½)	Low-mercury fish, such as salmon, skipjack or chunk-light tuna, halibut, cod, or mahi-mahi (3 to 5 ounces)	Olive, avocado, or coconut oil (1 tablespoon)	
Whole-grain bread (1 slice)	Shellfish such as shrimp, crab, or lobster (4 ounces)	Olives (5 to 8)	
Whole-wheat tortilla (1, 6-inch)	Whole eggs (1 or 2)		

* Keep in mind that many foods and beverages contain a combination of carbs, fat, and protein. However, in this table, each food is listed under the category it is most commonly associated with.
† Parenthetical amounts are equal to one serving.

FOODS TO EAT IN MODERATION

CARBS* (PROVIDES ~15 GRAMS OF CARBS/SERVING)	PROTEINS	FATS	BEVERAGES
Banana (½, medium size)†	Fatty cuts of meat (3 ounces)	Vegetable oils, such as canola, safflower, sunflower, corn, or soybean oil (no more than 1 tablespoon)	Cow's milk (8 ounces)
Fruit (cut), such as pineapple, watermelon, grapes, or melon (½ cup)	Soymilk, unsweetened (1 cup)		Juice (no more than 4 ounces)
Breakfast cereals (½ cup)	Turkey bacon, low-sodium (1 or 2 strips)		
Condiments, such as ketchup, barbecue sauce, mayonnaise, or mustard (1 tablespoon)			
Dried fruit (no more than ¼ cup)			
Natural sweeteners, such as maple syrup or honey (no more than 1 tablespoon)			
Whole-wheat crackers or pita chips (1 serving)			

*Keep in mind that many foods and beverages contain a combination of carbs, fat, and protein. However, in this table, each food is listed under the category it is most commonly associated with.
† Parenthetical amounts are equal to one serving.

CARBS	PROTEINS	FATS	BEVERAGES
Pastries	High-mercury fish, such as swordfish, shark, tilefish, king mackerel, albacore tuna, or marlin	Products made with hydrogenated or partially hydrogenated oils, such as margarine	Alcohol
Refined grains, such as white bread, white rice, white pasta, or anything made from white flour (limit as much as possible)	Processed deli meats and sausages	Trans fat	Caffeinated drinks
Granola bars, pretzels, or chips (limit as much as possible)	Raw eggs		Sweetened or processed coffee creamers
	Raw or undercooked meats		
	Highly processed cheeses (limit as much as possible)		

‡ *In addition to the foods in this table, I recommend avoiding "diet" foods and those made with artificial sweeteners, including aspartame, sucralose, and saccharin, which are made of chemicals and can encourage sugar cravings and dependence. Stevia is a natural and much safer no-calorie sweetener option to be used in moderation, as needed.*

The Basics of Portion Control

Now that you have a better understanding of healthy sources of carbohydrates, proteins, and fats, it is also important to have a good grasp on what a proper portion looks like. Practicing portion control is the key to keeping carbohydrate intake in check and managing blood sugar levels. When using the recipes in this book, remember to pay particular attention to the serving size and measurements, since these are the exact portions to follow to control blood sugar levels.

The good news is you don't need to have fancy equipment to measure your food. While measuring cups and spoons are helpful in your home kitchen, you may not have access to them when you are away from home or at a restaurant. In that case, use the "No-Brainer Guide to Portions" for help determining the proper portion size of commonly consumed foods.

NO-BRAINER GUIDE TO PORTIONS

SERVING SIZE	VISUAL REFERENCE
1 teaspoon	1 die
1 tablespoon	Poker chip or your thumb
2 tablespoons	Golf ball
¼ cup	One level handful
½ cup	A computer mouse
1 cup	Baseball or your fist
4 ounces meat, fish, or poultry	Deck of cards or your palm
1 ounce	Four dice or a string cheese stick

The Plate Method

The plate method provides an easy visual reference for managing portion sizes. Fill ½ of a roughly 9-inch plate with nonstarchy vegetables, ¼ with high-quality proteins, and ¼ with complex and high-fiber carbohydrates. Remember to include a healthy fat, which can be a healthy cooking oil or a garnish like sliced avocado.

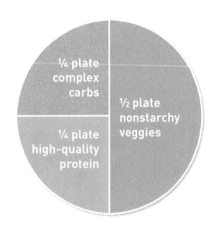

Be Careful of Skipping or Skimping on Meals

Although pregnancy may make you more aware of your changing body size and weight, skipping meals or strict dieting should be avoided. Pregnancy is a time of increased nutritional needs for mother and baby and requires specific and balanced nutrition.

This meal plan promotes a minimum of three meals per day to maximize nutrient intake and manage blood sugar levels to prevent hypoglycemia (low blood sugar) and hyperglycemia (high blood sugar).

In addition to eating three balanced meals, smart snacking is a healthy way to manage your blood sugar. Snacks can help you manage hunger and prevent low blood sugar levels caused by going too long without eating. Knowing you can have a snack also discourages overeating at mealtimes, which can cause blood sugar to rise too high. In general, snacks should be eaten 2 to 3 hours after the previous meal but not within 1 to 2 hours of your next meal. Snacks should have 15 grams or fewer carbohydrates and contain a healthy source of protein, fat, or both. The snack options in the next chapter offer examples of balanced snacks.

POSTPARTUM & BEYOND PREGNANCY

After your baby arrives, you may still have questions about your blood sugar. The good news is gestational diabetes resolves in about 90 percent of women after birth. However, women who have had gestational diabetes are more likely to develop it during future pregnancies and about seven times more likely to develop diabetes later in life, so postpartum follow-up with a physician is crucial.

Though it may be tempting to take a break from your structured meal plan, eating at least three healthy, balanced meals per day that include complex carbohydrates, protein, and fat is critical to lowering your risk of postpartum complications. It is also a good idea to continue checking your blood sugar levels for at least a few weeks after birth and to discuss the results with your physician. Gradually losing weight, breastfeeding, and being physically active are also excellent ways to stay healthy and maintain the endurance you need to give your best self to your baby.

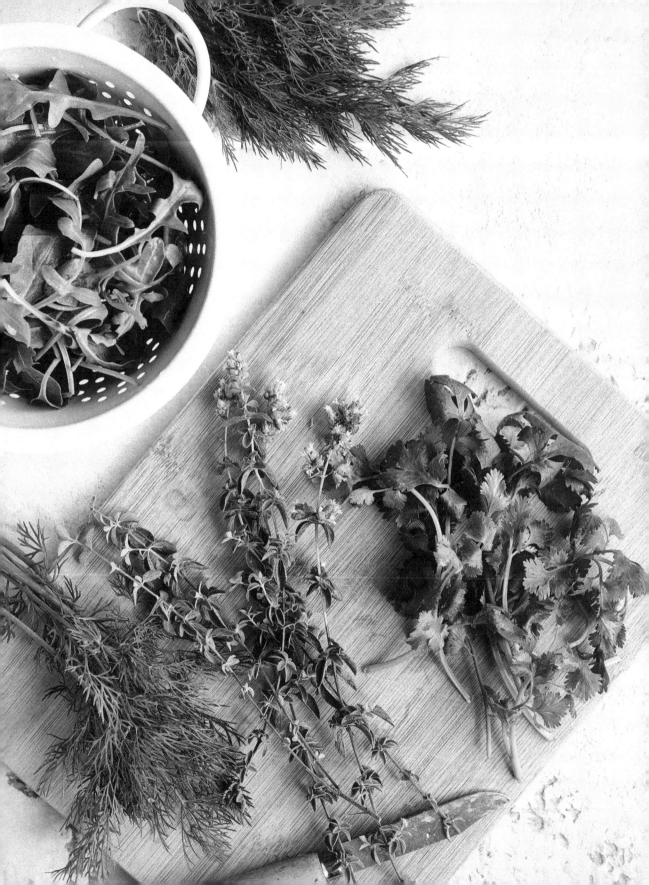

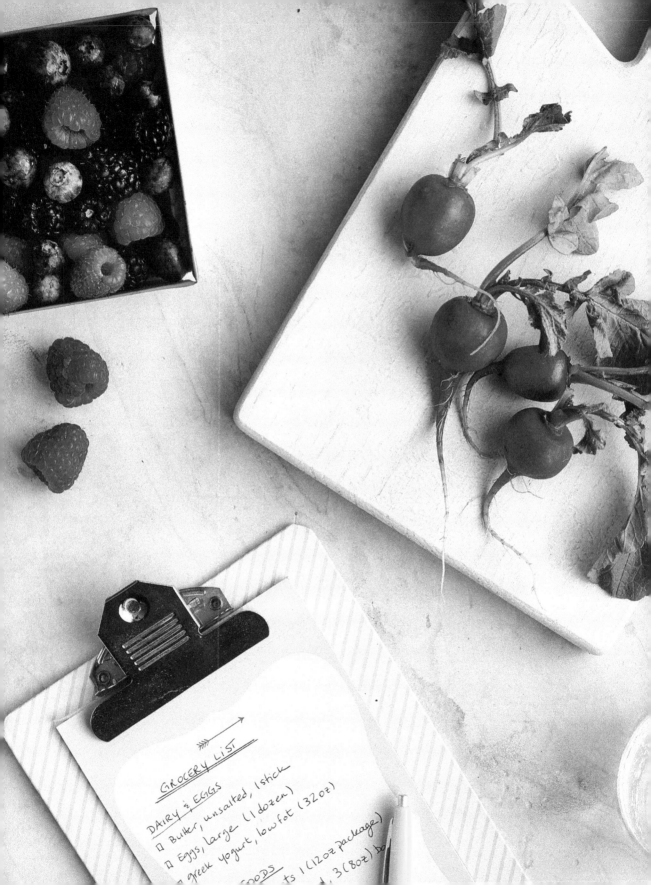

GROCERY LIST →

<u>DAIRY & EGGS</u>
☐ Butter, unsalted, 1 stick
☐ Eggs, large (1 dozen)
☐ greek yogurt, lowfat (32oz)

_OODS
ts 1 (12oz package)
d, 3 (8oz) bo

CHAPTER TWO

The 4-Week Meal Plan

The meal plan allows you to take control of your health quickly by eliminating the worry and guesswork from meal planning. Designed with an understanding that you lead a busy life, the meal plan frequently incorporates leftovers, so you do not need to cook three times a day. Weekday breakfasts and lunches are designed to be simple, grab-and-go meals. Dinners do require some prep work, but many can be made in under 30 minutes, and most require fewer than 10 ingredients. Note that the chapters that follow purposefully include more recipes than appear in the meal plan to provide variety and accommodate your personal preferences.

If you're new to following a meal plan, the idea may seem daunting. But don't let that fear keep you from trying—simply do the best you can, and don't be too hard on yourself if you don't have time to cook one day. Here are a few tips that can help:

» **Plan ahead.** Schedule meal preparation into your calendar as you would an appointment. On nights you won't be home to cook, put a meal in the slow cooker that morning, or prepare a larger meal earlier in the week so you'll have leftovers.

» **Batch cook.** Intentionally cook large portions (double or triple batches) of things like whole grains, hardboiled eggs, and meats, so they are ready to use when you need them.

» **Keep a prepared kitchen.** Stock staples and go-to items in your pantry. Chop vegetables ahead of time and store them in sealed containers in the refrigerator.

» **Be ready with backup.** Keep a list of your favorite quick and easy meals, and stock those ingredients in your pantry in case you unavoidably run out of time to go shopping.

Week 1

The first week of starting any new program is always the hardest. This week, focus on the results you will see in your blood sugar levels and your overall health. New portion sizes, new flavors, a new eating schedule, and possibly putting in more time in the kitchen may require some adjustments, but keep at it. Use the notes sections to keep track of your progress, favorite recipes, substitutions, and personal preferences.

WEEK 1 MEAL PREP TIPS

Prepare these recipes and ingredients over the weekend—or whatever day fits your schedule—to save time during the week:

» Make Blueberry Coconut Breakfast Cookies (page 47)

» Wash and chop Brussels sprouts for Salmon with Brussels Sprouts (page 133)

» Hardboil 6 large eggs

» Cook 1 cup brown rice or quinoa to last for the week (makes 2½ to 3 cups cooked rice or quinoa)

» Prepare tuna mixture for Open-Faced Tuna Melts (page 78)

» Make Thai-Style Peanut Sauce (page 145)

» Prep vegetables for Ratatouille (page 86)

Week 1 Snack Options

» ½ cup plain low-fat Greek yogurt topped with 1 teaspoon honey and 1 to 2 tablespoons nuts

» ½ to 1 cup shelled edamame

» 1 ounce 70% or greater dark chocolate

» ½ cup berries + ¼ cup nuts of choice

» ½ cup baby carrots (or other veggie sticks) with ¼ cup hummus

» 1 string cheese + ¼ cup nuts of choice (or ½ cup berries)

» Leftover Blueberry Coconut Breakfast Cookies

MONDAY

BREAKFAST	Blueberry Coconut Breakfast Cookies + 1 to 2 hardboiled eggs (29g carbs)
SNACK	½ cup plain low-fat Greek yogurt topped with 1 teaspoon honey and 1 to 2 tablespoons nuts (13g carbs)
LUNCH	Open-Faced Tuna Melts + ½ cup berries (34g carbs)
SNACK	½ cup shelled edamame (7g carbs)
DINNER	Salmon with Brussels Sprouts + ½ cup cooked brown rice or quinoa (35g carbs)
SNACK	1 ounce 70% or greater dark chocolate (13g carbs)
TOTAL CARBS	131g carbs

Notes

TUESDAY

BREAKFAST	Tropical Greek Yogurt Bowl (21g carbs)
SNACK	½ cup berries + ¼ cup nuts of choice (15g carbs)
LUNCH	Leftover Salmon with Brussels Sprouts + ½ cup brown rice or quinoa (35g carbs)
SNACK	½ serving leftover Open-Faced Tuna Melts (14g carbs)
DINNER	Greek Chicken Stuffed Peppers + Ratatouille (44g carbs)
SNACK	½ cup baby carrots with ¼ cup hummus (15g carbs)
TOTAL CARBS	144g carbs

Notes

WEDNESDAY

BREAKFAST	Leftover Blueberry Coconut Breakfast Cookies + 1 to 2 hardboiled eggs (29g carbs)
SNACK	½ serving leftover Open-Faced Tuna Melts (14g carbs)
LUNCH	Leftover Greek Chicken Stuffed Peppers + leftover Ratatouille (44g carbs)
SNACK	1 cup shelled edamame (14g carbs)
DINNER	Tuna Casserole + Italian Zucchini Boats (32g carbs)
SNACK	1 string cheese + ¼ cup nuts of choice (9g carbs)
TOTAL CARBS	142g carbs

Notes

THURSDAY

BREAKFAST	Leftover Tropical Greek Yogurt Bowl (21g carbs)
SNACK	1 string cheese + ¼ cup nuts of choice (9g carbs)
LUNCH	Leftover Tuna Casserole + leftover Italian Zucchini Boats (32g carbs)
SNACK	2 leftover Blueberry Coconut Breakfast Cookies (19g carbs)
DINNER	Smothered Burritos + ½ cup baby carrots with ¼ cup hummus (45g carbs
SNACK	1 ounce 70% or greater dark chocolate (13g carbs)
TOTAL CARBS	143g carbs

Notes

FRIDAY

BREAKFAST	Leftover Blueberry Coconut Breakfast Cookies + 1 to 2 hardboiled eggs (29g carbs)
SNACK	1 string cheese + ¼ cup nuts of choice (9g carbs)
LUNCH	Leftover Smothered Burritos (30g carbs)
SNACK	½ cup plain low-fat Greek yogurt topped with 1 teaspoon honey and 1 to 2 tablespoons nuts (13g carbs)
DINNER	Edamame Peanut Bowl + ½ cup veggie sticks with ¼ cup hummus (42g carbs)
SNACK	1 ounce 70% or greater dark chocolate (13g carbs)
TOTAL CARBS	136g carbs

Notes

SATURDAY

BREAKFAST	Brussels Sprouts and Egg Scramble + 1 small whole fruit (30g carbs)
SNACK	½ cup berries + ¼ cup nuts of choice (15g carbs)
LUNCH	Leftover Edamame Peanut Bowl (27g carbs)
SNACK	½ cup baby carrots with ¼ cup hummus (15g carbs)
DINNER	Baked Turkey Spaghetti + 2 servings leftover Ratatouille (42g carbs)
SNACK	½ cup plain low-fat Greek yogurt topped with 1 teaspoon honey and 1 to 2 tablespoons nuts (13g carbs)
TOTAL CARBS	142g carbs

Notes

WEEK 1

SUNDAY

BREAKFAST	Leftover Brussels Sprouts and Egg Scramble + 1 small whole fruit (30g carbs)
SNACK	½ cup plain low-fat Greek yogurt topped with 1 teaspoon honey and 1 to 2 tablespoons nuts (13g carbs)
LUNCH	Leftover Baked Turkey Spaghetti + 1 cup shelled edamame (26g carbs)
SNACK	½ cup baby carrots with ¼ cup hummus (15g carbs)
DINNER	Chicken Tender and Brussels Sprout Cobb Salad (34g carbs)
SNACK	1 ounce 70% or greater dark chocolate (13g carbs)
TOTAL CARBS	131g carbs

Notes

WEEK 1 SHOPPING LIST

Canned and Bottled Items

» Chickpeas, low-sodium, 1 (15-ounce) can
» Spaghetti sauce, 1 (24-ounce) jar
» Tomatoes, diced, no salt added, 1 (15-ounce) can
» Tuna, chunk light, 4 (5-ounce) cans

Dairy and Eggs

» Butter, unsalted (1 stick)
» Cheddar cheese, shredded (1 pound)
» Eggs, large (1½ dozen)
» Feta, crumbled (6 ounces)
» Greek yogurt, plain low-fat, 1 (32-ounce) container
» Parmesan cheese, shredded (5 ounces)
» String cheese, 1 (12-ounce) package

Frozen Foods

» Broccoli, florets, 1 (10- to 12-ounce) package
» Cauliflower, florets, 1 (10- to 12-ounce) package
» Edamame, shelled, 3 (8-ounce) bags

Meat and Fish

» Chicken, 4 (4-ounce) boneless, skinless breasts
» Chicken, tenders (1 pound)
» Salmon, 4 (4-ounce) skinless fillets

» Turkey, ground, 93% lean
(2 pounds)

» Turkey bacon, low-sodium,
1 (12-ounce) package

Pantry Items

» Almond milk, unsweetened
» Avocado oil cooking spray
» Black pepper
» Chia seeds
» Chicken broth, low-sodium
» Coconut flakes,
dried, unsweetened
» Coconut flour
» Cranberries, dried
» English muffins, 100% whole
wheat, 1 (12-ounce) package
» Garlic powder
» Honey
» Honey mustard
» Hot sauce (optional)
» Nuts of choice
» Oil, extra-virgin olive
» Oil, sesame
» Onion powder
» Oregano, dried
» Paprika, smoked
» Peanut butter, natural
» Rice, brown (or quinoa)
» Salsa
» Salt
» Soy sauce, low-sodium
» Thyme, dried
» Tortillas, yellow corn, taco size,
1 (16-ounce) package
» Vanilla extract
» Vinegar, rice

» Walnuts
» Whole-wheat flour

Produce

» Baby carrots or other veggie
sticks, 1 (1-pound) package
» Bananas (2)
» Bell pepper, green (1)
» Bell peppers, red (3)
» Berries of choice, fresh (8 ounces)
» Blueberries, fresh or frozen
(8 ounces)
» Broccoli, florets, 1 (10- to
12-ounce) package
» Brussels sprouts, shaved,
2 (9-ounce) packages
» Brussels sprouts, whole (2 pounds)
» Carrot noodles,
2 (10-ounce) packages
» Eggplant (1)
» Fruit of choice, small (2)
» Ginger, small piece (1)
» Kiwis (4)
» Lemon (1)
» Limes (2)
» Onions, yellow (2)
» Zucchini (3)
» Zucchini noodles,
2 (10-ounce) packages

Other

» Applesauce, unsweetened,
1 (24-ounce) container
» Chocolate, dark, 70% or greater
(4 ounces)
» Hummus, 1 (10-ounce) container

Week 2

As you head into week 2, you will continue to notice improvements in your blood sugar levels, and by now your taste buds are getting used to new foods and flavors. You may also notice how satisfying foods are when the three macronutrients are balanced.

Keep in mind that this meal plan is not a "diet." It is a plan that helps you make sure you're giving your body the nutrients it needs to sustain a healthy pregnancy, while strategically balancing your carbohydrate intake. Because the meal plans don't include beverages, be sure you are staying hydrated.

WEEK 2 MEAL PREP TIPS

» Make Orange Muffins (page 49)
» Dice vegetables for Maple Sausage Frittata (page 57)
» Chop vegetables for Steak Fajita Bake (page 119) and Veggie Fajitas (page 83)

WEEK 2 SNACK OPTIONS

» 2 cups air-popped popcorn tossed with 2 tablespoons unsalted peanuts
» ¼ cup unsalted trail mix (no chocolate chips)
» 5 to 10 whole-wheat crackers topped with 2 tablespoons low-fat cream cheese
» ½ pear, sliced and sprinkled with cinnamon, or ½ cup grapes + 1 string cheese
» ½ cup plain low-fat Greek yogurt topped with 1 teaspoon honey (or maple syrup) and 2 tablespoons berries
» Leftover Orange Muffins

MONDAY

BREAKFAST	2 Orange Muffins (32g carbs)
SNACK	5 to 10 whole-wheat crackers with 2 tablespoons low-fat cream cheese (18g carbs)
LUNCH	Open-Faced Chicken and Onion Grilled Cheese + ¼ cup grapes (28g carbs)
SNACK	¼ cup unsalted trail mix (17g carbs)
DINNER	Steak Fajita Bake + 1 cup steamed broccoli (37g carbs)
SNACK	½ pear, sliced and sprinkled with cinnamon + 1 string cheese (15g carbs)
TOTAL CARBS	149g carbs

Notes

TUESDAY

BREAKFAST	Crepe Cakes + Maple Sausage Frittata (25g carbs)
SNACK	1 leftover Orange Muffin (16g carbs)
LUNCH	Leftover Steak Fajita Bake + 1 cup steamed broccoli (37g carbs)
SNACK	½ cup plain low-fat Greek yogurt with 1 teaspoon honey and 2 tablespoons berries (13g carbs)
DINNER	Chickpea Coconut Curry + Chicken Salad Salad (40g carbs)
SNACK	2 cups air-popped popcorn with 2 tablespoons unsalted peanuts (15g carbs)
TOTAL CARBS	148g carbs

Notes

WEDNESDAY

BREAKFAST	2 leftover Orange Muffins (32g carbs)
SNACK	Leftover Crepe Cakes (15g carbs)
LUNCH	Leftover Open-Faced Chicken and Onion Grilled Cheese + ¼ cup grapes (28g carbs)
SNACK	½ pear, sliced and sprinkled with cinnamon + 1 string cheese (15g carbs)
DINNER	Fish Tacos + Cauliflower Steaks (42g carbs)
SNACK	5 to 10 whole-wheat crackers with 2 tablespoons low-fat cream cheese (18g carbs)
TOTAL CARBS	150g carbs

Notes

THURSDAY

BREAKFAST	Leftover Crepe Cakes + leftover Maple Sausage Frittata (25g carbs)
SNACK	¼ cup unsalted trail mix (17g carbs)
LUNCH	Leftover Chickpea Coconut Curry + leftover Chicken Salad Salad (40g carbs)
SNACK	1 leftover Orange Muffin (16g carbs)
DINNER	Creamy Garlic Chicken with Broccoli + leftover Cauliflower Steak (40g carbs)
SNACK	½ cup plain low-fat Greek yogurt with 1 teaspoon honey and 2 tablespoons berries (13g carbs)
TOTAL CARBS	151g carbs

Notes

FRIDAY

BREAKFAST	Peanut Butter Power Oats (27g carbs)
SNACK	½ cup plain low-fat Greek yogurt with 1 teaspoon honey and 2 tablespoons berries (13g carbs)
LUNCH	Leftover Fish Tacos (28g carbs)
SNACK	5 to 10 whole-wheat crackers with 2 tablespoons low-fat cream cheese (18g carbs)
DINNER	Leftover Creamy Garlic Chicken with Broccoli + leftover Cauliflower Steaks (40g carbs)
SNACK	1 leftover Orange Muffin (16g carbs)
TOTAL CARBS	142g carbs

Notes

SATURDAY

BREAKFAST	Leftover Crepe Cakes + leftover Maple Sausage Frittata (25g carbs)
SNACK	1 leftover Orange Muffin (16g carbs)
LUNCH	Veggie Fajitas (37g carbs)
SNACK	¼ cup unsalted trail mix (17g carbs)
DINNER	One-Pan Chicken Dinner (37g carbs)
SNACK	2 cups air-popped popcorn with 2 tablespoons unsalted peanuts (15g carbs)
TOTAL CARBS	147g carbs

Notes

WEEK 2

SUNDAY

BREAKFAST	Leftover Peanut Butter Power Oats (27g carbs)
SNACK	5 to 10 whole-wheat crackers with 2 tablespoons low-fat cream cheese (18g carbs)
LUNCH	Leftover Veggie Fajitas (37g carbs)
SNACK	½ cup plain low-fat Greek yogurt with 1 teaspoon honey and 2 tablespoons berries (13g carbs)
DINNER	Leftover One-Pan Chicken Dinner (37g carbs)
SNACK	½ cup grapes + 1 string cheese (15g carbs)
TOTAL CARBS	147g carbs

Notes

WEEK 2 SHOPPING LIST

Canned and Bottled Items

- » Black beans, low-sodium, 1 (15-ounce) can
- » Chickpeas, low-sodium, 1 (15-ounce) can
- » Coconut milk, 1 (15-ounce) can

Dairy and Eggs

- » Butter, unsalted (1 stick)
- » Cream cheese, plain, reduced-fat, 1 (8-ounce) package
- » Eggs, large (1½ dozen)
- » Greek yogurt, plain, low-fat, 1 (32-ounce) container
- » Half-and-half (1 pint)
- » Provolone or Swiss cheese, 1 (8-ounce) package
- » String cheese, 1 (12-ounce) package

Meat and Fish

- » Chicken, 8 (4-ounce) breasts
- » Chicken or turkey breakfast sausage links, maple-flavored, 1 (6- to 10-ounce) package
- » Chicken, rotisserie (1 whole)
- » Cod, 4 (6-ounce) fillets
- » Steak, sirloin (10 ounces)

Pantry Items

- » Almond flour
- » Almond milk, unsweetened
- » Avocado oil cooking spray
- » Baking powder
- » Black pepper

- » Bread, 100% whole-wheat
- » Cardamom, ground
- » Chia seeds
- » Chili powder
- » Cinnamon, ground
- » Crackers, whole-wheat,
  1 (6- to 8-ounce) box
- » Cumin, ground
- » Curry powder
- » Garlic powder
- » Ginger, ground
- » Honey
- » Honey mustard
- » Italian seasoning
- » Mayonnaise, low-fat
- » Oats, rolled
- » Oil, avocado
- » Oil, extra-virgin olive
- » Oil, olive
- » Onion powder
- » Peanuts, unsalted
- » Peanut butter, natural
- » Pecans (optional)
- » Popcorn, air-popped,
  1 small package
- » Rice, brown (or quinoa)
- » Salt
- » Tortillas, 100% whole-wheat, soft taco size, 1 (16-ounce) package
- » Tortillas, yellow corn, soft taco size, 1 (16-ounce) package
- » Tortillas, yellow corn, street taco size, 1 (11- to 12-ounce) package
- » Trail mix, unsalted (4 ounces)
- » Vanilla extract
- » Vinegar, red wine
- » Walnut pieces (optional)

Produce

- » Arugula, 1 (5-ounce) bag
- » Avocados (3)
- » Bananas (2)
- » Bell peppers, green (3)
- » Bell peppers, red (3)
- » Bell pepper, yellow (1)
- » Berries of choice, fresh or frozen (10 ounces)
- » Broccoli, florets, 2 (12-ounce) packages
- » Brussels sprouts, whole (1 pound)
- » Cabbage, shredded, 1 (10-ounce) package
- » Cauliflower (2 heads)
- » Cilantro, fresh (1 bunch)
- » Grapes, red, seedless (8-ounce)
- » Lemon (1)
- » Lettuce, romaine (1 head)
- » Lime (1)
- » Onions, white (2)
- » Onion, yellow (1)
- » Orange (1)
- » Pear (1)
- » Portobello mushrooms, sliced, 1 (8-ounce) package
- » Spinach, fresh, 1 (16-ounce) bag
- » Sweet potatoes, cubed, 1 (10-ounce) package
- » Tomato (1)
- » Tomatoes, cherry, 1 (10-ounce) package

Week 3

This week is a good time to check in with yourself about the changes you have experienced. Have you noticed your cravings for sweets decrease? Or perhaps your energy levels have improved, or you have discovered that you are needing less food to keep you full than before? Share these findings with both yourself and a loved one, or even consider writing them down to help you remember and be accountable. Even if you haven't followed your meal plan exactly, it's okay. Progress, and not perfection, is what matters most.

WEEK 3 MEAL PREP TIPS

» Make Roasted Red Pepper Spread (page 142)
» Make Simple Grain-Free Biscuits (page 48)
» Slice cucumber and onion for Open-Faced Greek Chicken Sandwiches (page 76)
» Hardboil 11 eggs for Farro Bowl (page 97) and snacks
» Mix ingredients for No-Tuna Lettuce Wraps (page 92)

WEEK 3 SNACK OPTIONS

» ½ medium-size apple topped with 1 tablespoon almond butter (tip: squeeze lemon juice over the other half of the apple and place it in an airtight bag or container to keep from browning)
» 1 slice whole-wheat toast topped with ¼ avocado, seasoned with freshly ground black pepper
» ½ cup low-fat cottage cheese topped with ¼ cup berries
» 5 to 10 pita chips (or whole-wheat crackers) dipped in ¼ cup guacamole
» 1 mandarin orange (or kiwi) + 1 hardboiled egg

MONDAY

BREAKFAST	Berry Almond Smoothie + Simple Grain-Free Biscuit (32g carbs)
SNACK	1 mandarin orange + 1 hardboiled egg (11g carbs)
LUNCH	Open-Faced Greek Chicken Sandwiches (25g carbs)
SNACK	1 slice whole-wheat toast with ¼ avocado and black pepper (18g carbs)
DINNER	Farro Bowl (42g carbs)
SNACK	½ cup low-fat cottage cheese with ¼ cup berries (9g carbs)
TOTAL CARBS	137g carbs

Notes

TUESDAY

BREAKFAST	Leftover Berry Almond Smoothie + leftover Simple Grain-Free Biscuit (32g carbs)
SNACK	½ apple with 1 tablespoon almond butter (16g carbs)
LUNCH	Leftover Open-Faced Greek Chicken Sandwiches (25g carbs)
SNACK	1 mandarin orange + 1 hardboiled egg (11g carbs)
DINNER	Roasted Pork Loin + Summer Salad (44g carbs)
SNACK	5 to 10 pita chips with ¼ cup guacamole (15g carbs)
TOTAL CARBS	143g carbs

Notes

WEDNESDAY

BREAKFAST	Loaded Avocado + leftover Simple Grain-Free Biscuit + ½ cup berries (30g carbs)
SNACK	1 mandarin orange + 1 hardboiled egg (11g carbs)
LUNCH	Leftover Farro Bowl (42g carbs)
SNACK	½ cup low-fat cottage cheese with ¼ cup berries (9g carbs)
DINNER	Peppered Chicken with Balsamic Kale + Stuffed Portobello Mushrooms + ¼ cup brown rice or quinoa (32g carbs)
SNACK	½ apple with 1 tablespoon almond butter (16g carbs)
TOTAL CARBS	140g carbs

Notes

THURSDAY

BREAKFAST	Leftover Berry Almond Smoothie + leftover Simple Grain-Free Biscuit (32g carbs)
SNACK	½ cup low-fat cottage cheese with ¼ cup berries (9g carbs)
LUNCH	Leftover Roasted Pork Loin + leftover Summer Salad (44g carbs)
SNACK	1 slice whole-wheat toast with ¼ avocado and black pepper (18g carbs)
DINNER	Leftover Peppered Chicken with Balsamic Kale + leftover Stuffed Portobello Mushrooms + ¼ cup brown rice or quinoa (32g carbs)
SNACK	1 mandarin orange + 1 hardboiled egg (11g carbs)
TOTAL CARBS	146g carbs

Notes

FRIDAY

BREAKFAST	Leftover Loaded Avocado + leftover Grain Free-Biscuit + ½ cup berries (30g carbs)
SNACK	½ apple with 1 tablespoon almond butter (16g carbs)
LUNCH	No-Tuna Lettuce Wraps (41g carbs)
SNACK	½ cup low-fat cottage cheese with ¼ cup berries (9g carbs)
DINNER	Catfish with Corn and Pepper Relish (41g carbs)
SNACK	1 mandarin orange + 1 hardboiled egg (11g carbs)
TOTAL CARBS	148g carbs

Notes

SATURDAY

BREAKFAST	Sausage, Sweet Potato, and Kale Hash (32g carbs)
SNACK	5 to 10 pita chips with ¼ cup guacamole (15g carbs)
LUNCH	Leftover No-Tuna Lettuce Wraps (41g carbs)
SNACK	½ cup low-fat cottage cheese with ¼ cup berries (9g carbs)
DINNER	Coconut Lime Chicken + Cauliflower Leek Soup (29g carbs)
SNACK	1 mandarin orange + 1 hardboiled egg (11g carbs)
TOTAL CARBS	137g carbs

Notes

SUNDAY

BREAKFAST	Leftover Sausage, Sweet Potato, and Kale Hash (32g carbs)
SNACK	½ apple with 1 tablespoon almond butter (16g carbs)
LUNCH	Leftover Coconut Lime Chicken + leftover Cauliflower Leek Soup (29g carbs)
SNACK	1 mandarin orange + 1 hardboiled egg (11g carbs)
DINNER	Leftover Catfish with Corn and Pepper Relish (41g carbs)
SNACK	1 slice whole-wheat toast with ¼ avocado and black pepper (18g carbs)
TOTAL CARBS	147g carbs

Notes

WEEK 3 SHOPPING LIST

Canned and Bottled Items

» Black beans, low-sodium, 1 (15-ounce) can
» Chickpeas, low-sodium, 2 (15-ounce) cans
» Coconut milk, unsweetened, 1 (15-ounce) can
» Red bell peppers, roasted, 1 (16-ounce) jar

Dairy and Eggs

» Butter, unsalted (1 stick)
» Cottage cheese, low-fat, 1 (16-ounce) container
» Greek yogurt, plain, low-fat, 1 (16-ounce) container
» Eggs, large (2 dozen)
» Feta, crumbled (6 ounces)
» Half-and-half (4 ounces)

Frozen Foods

» Berries of choice, 1 (24-ounce) bag
» Corn, 1 (10-ounce) bag

Meat and Fish

» Catfish, 4 (5-ounce) fillets
» Chicken, 8 (4-ounce) boneless, skinless breasts
» Chicken or turkey breakfast sausage links, 1 (8-ounce) package
» Chicken, rotisserie (½)
» Pork loin (1 pound)

Pantry Items

» Almond butter, natural
» Almond flour
» Almond milk, unsweetened, vanilla
» Avocado oil cooking spray
» Black pepper
» Bread, 100% whole-wheat
» Cumin, ground
» Farro
» Garlic powder
» Honey
» Honey mustard
» Oil, coconut
» Oil, extra-virgin olive
» Pita chips or whole-wheat crackers, 1 (6- to 8-ounce) box
» Red pepper flakes
» Rice, brown (or quinoa)
» Rosemary, dried
» Salt
» Tahini, unsalted
» Vegetable broth, low-sodium
» Vinegar, apple cider
» Vinegar, balsamic
» Walnuts

Produce

» Apples (2)
» Asparagus (1 bunch)
» Arugula, 2 (5-ounce) bags
» Avocados (4)
» Bell peppers, red (3)
» Carrots (4)
» Cauliflower, florets, 1 (12-ounce) package
» Celery (1 bunch)
» Cilantro, fresh (1 bunch)
» Cucumber (1)
» Garlic, whole or minced
» Scallions (1 bunch)
» Jalapeño pepper (1)
» Kale (4 bunches)
» Leeks (3)
» Lemons (2)
» Lettuce, butter or romaine (1 head)
» Limes (3)
» Mixed greens, 1 (16-ounce) bag
» Onion, red (1)
» Oranges, mandarin (or kiwi) (7)
» Peaches (2)
» Portobello mushrooms, whole caps (8)
» Potatoes, gold (2)
» Spinach, fresh, 1 (16-ounce) bag
» Sweet potatoes, cubed, 1 (10-ounce) package
» Tomatoes, cherry, 1 (10-ounce) package

Other

» Red pepper hummus, 1 (8-ounce) container
» Guacamole, 1 (8-ounce) container

Week 4

Congratulations! You made it to week 4. You've completed 21 days of healthier eating and balanced blood sugar levels, and that is huge. I hope that by now you have discovered some of your favorite meals and foods. Celebrate your efforts and success so far, and remember that finishing this 4-week meal plan is not the end, but rather a new starting point on your health journey. Keep up the excellent work!

WEEK 4 MEAL PREP TIPS

» Make a double batch of Creamy Avocado Dressing (page 139) and one batch of Creamy Dill Dressing (page 140)

» Chop bell peppers for Breakfast Tacos (page 53)

» Prepare and cook all vegetables for Roasted Vegetables with Creamy Dill Dressing (page 85)

WEEK 4 SNACK OPTIONS

» 1 string cheese paired with ¼ cup almonds (or other nuts)

» 1 ounce 70% or greater dark chocolate

» ½ cup shelled edamame

» 2 cups air-popped popcorn tossed with 2 tablespoons unsalted peanuts

» ¼ cup unsalted trail mix (no chocolate chips)

» ½ cup baby carrots (or other veggie sticks) dipped in ¼ cup hummus

MONDAY

BREAKFAST	Huevos Rancheros Remix + ½ cup berries (24g carbs)
SNACK	½ cup baby carrots with ¼ cup hummus (15g carbs)
LUNCH	Roasted Vegetables with Creamy Dill Dressing + 4 ounces grilled chicken breast (optional) (38g carbs)
SNACK	¼ cup unsalted trail mix (17g carbs)
DINNER	Sloppy Joes (36g carbs)
SNACK	1 ounce 70% or greater dark chocolate (13g carbs)
TOTAL CARBS	143g carbs

Notes

TUESDAY

BREAKFAST	Leftover Huevos Rancheros Remix + ½ cup berries (24g carbs)
SNACK	1 string cheese + ¼ cup almonds (9g carbs)
LUNCH	Leftover Roasted Vegetables with Creamy Dill Dressing + 4 ounces grilled chicken breast (optional) (38g carbs)
SNACK	½ cup baby carrots with ¼ cup hummus (15g carbs)
DINNER	Shrimp Stir-Fry + ½ cup shelled edamame (35g carbs)
SNACK	2 cups air-popped popcorn with 2 tablespoons unsalted peanuts (15g carbs)
TOTAL CARBS	136g carbs

Notes

WEDNESDAY

BREAKFAST	Breakfast Tacos (28g carbs)
SNACK	1 string cheese + ¼ cup almonds (9g carbs)
LUNCH	Leftover Sloppy Joes (36g carbs)
SNACK	¼ cup unsalted trail mix (17g carbs)
DINNER	Cauli-Flowing Sweet Potato + 4 ounces grilled chicken breast (36g carbs)
SNACK	1 ounce 70% or greater dark chocolate (13g carbs)
TOTAL CARBS	139g carbs

Notes

THURSDAY

BREAKFAST	Leftover Huevos Rancheros Remix + ½ cup berries (24g carbs)
SNACK	½ cup baby carrots with ¼ cup hummus (15g carbs)
LUNCH	Leftover Shrimp Stir-Fry + ½ cup shelled edamame (35g carbs)
SNACK	1 string cheese + ¼ cup almonds (9g carbs)
DINNER	Leftover Cauli-Flowing Sweet Potato + 4 ounces grilled chicken breast (36g carbs)
SNACK	2 cups air-popped popcorn with 2 tablespoons unsalted peanuts (15g carbs)
TOTAL CARBS	134g carbs

Notes

FRIDAY

BREAKFAST	Leftover Breakfast Tacos (28g carbs)
SNACK	1 string cheese + ¼ cup almonds (9g carbs)
LUNCH	Leftover Sloppy Joes (36g carbs)
SNACK	¼ cup unsalted trail mix (17g carbs)
DINNER	Creamy Cod with Asparagus + Mushroom and Cauliflower Rice Risotto (32g carbs)
SNACK	1 ounce 70% or greater dark chocolate (13g carbs)
TOTAL CARBS	135g carbs

Notes

SATURDAY

BREAKFAST	Coconut Pancakes topped with 1 cup berries (22g carbs)
SNACK	½ cup shelled edamame (7g carbs)
LUNCH	Leftover Creamy Cod with Asparagus + leftover Mushroom and Cauliflower Rice Risotto (32g carbs)
SNACK	½ cup baby carrots with ¼ cup hummus (15g carbs)
DINNER	Southwest Salad (41g carbs)
SNACK	2 cups air-popped popcorn with 2 tablespoons unsalted peanuts (15g carbs)
TOTAL CARBS	132g carbs

Notes

SUNDAY

BREAKFAST	Leftover Coconut Pancakes topped with 1 cup berries (22g carbs)
SNACK	1 string cheese + ¼ cup almonds (9g carbs)
LUNCH	Leftover Southwest Salad (41g carbs)
SNACK	¼ cup unsalted trail mix (17g carbs)
DINNER	Lazy Sushi + ½ cup shelled edamame (35g carbs)
SNACK	1 ounce 70% or greater dark chocolate (13g carbs)
TOTAL CARBS	137g carbs

Notes

WEEK 4 SHOPPING LIST

Canned and Bottled Items

» Black beans, low-sodium, 2 (15-ounce) cans
» Tomato sauce, no salt added, 1 (15-ounce) can
» Salsa verde, 1 (16-ounce) jar

Dairy and Eggs

» Cheddar cheese, sharp, shredded (8 ounces)
» Eggs, large (2 dozen)
» Greek yogurt, plain low-fat, 1 (16-ounce) container
» Half-and-half (12 ounces)
» Parmesan cheese, shredded (4 ounces)
» String cheese, 1 (12-ounce) package

Frozen Foods

» Broccoli, florets, 2 (10-ounce) packages
» Stir-fry vegetable mix, 2 (20-ounce) bags
» Edamame, shelled, 1 (8-ounce) bag

Meat and Fish

» Beef, ground, 93% lean (1 pound)
» Chicken, 8 (4-ounce) boneless, skinless breasts (2 optional)
» Cod, 4 (4-ounce) fillets
» Shrimp, medium, fresh, peeled and deveined (12 ounces)

Pantry Items

- » Almonds or nuts of choice
- » Almond milk, unsweetened
- » Avocado oil cooking spray
- » Baking powder
- » Black pepper
- » Chicken broth, low-sodium
- » Cinnamon, ground
- » Coconut flour
- » Cornstarch
- » Garlic powder
- » Ginger, ground
- » Honey
- » Hot sauce
- » Ketchup, no salt or sugar added
- » Mayonnaise, low-fat
- » Oil, extra-virgin olive
- » Oil, olive
- » Oil, sesame
- » Peanuts, unsalted
- » Popcorn, air-popped, 1 (4-ounce) bag
- » Rice, brown (or quinoa)
- » Salt
- » Sandwich thins, 100% whole-wheat
- » Soy sauce, low-sodium
- » Trail mix, unsalted
- » Tortillas, 100% whole-wheat, street taco size, 1 (11-ounce) package
- » Vanilla extract
- » Vinegar, rice
- » Worcestershire sauce, reduced-sodium

Produce

- » Avocados (4)
- » Asparagus (1 bunch)
- » Baby carrots or other veggie sticks, 1 (16-ounce) package
- » Bell pepper, green (1)
- » Bell peppers, red (2)
- » Berries of choice (24 ounces)
- » Brussels sprouts, whole (8 ounces)
- » Cabbage, shredded, 1 (10-ounce) bag
- » Cauliflower, florets, 2 (12-ounce) packages
- » Cauliflower rice, 2 (12-ounce) packages
- » Cilantro, fresh (2 bunches)
- » Cucumber (1)
- » Dill, fresh (1 bunch)
- » Lemon (1)
- » Limes (4)
- » Mixed greens, 2 (16-ounce) bags
- » Onion, yellow (1)
- » Portobello mushrooms, sliced 1 (8-ounce) package
- » Scallions (1 bunch)
- » Spinach, fresh, 1 (16-ounce) bag
- » Sweet potatoes (5)
- » Zucchini (1)

Other

- » Chocolate, dark, 70% or greater (4 ounces)
- » Hummus, 1 (8-ounce) container
- » Nori, dried, 2 (4-gram) packages

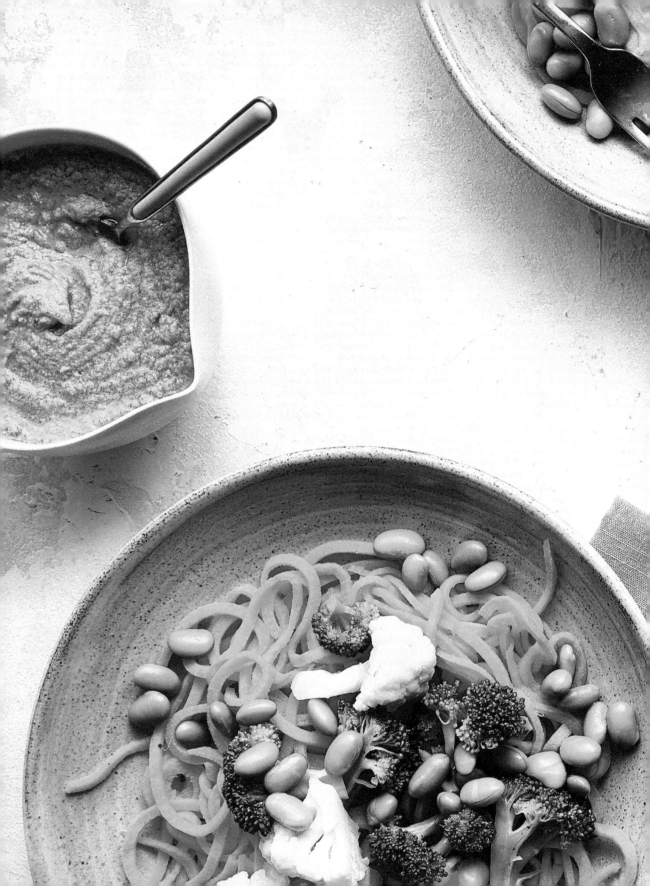

PART
2

THE
RECIPES

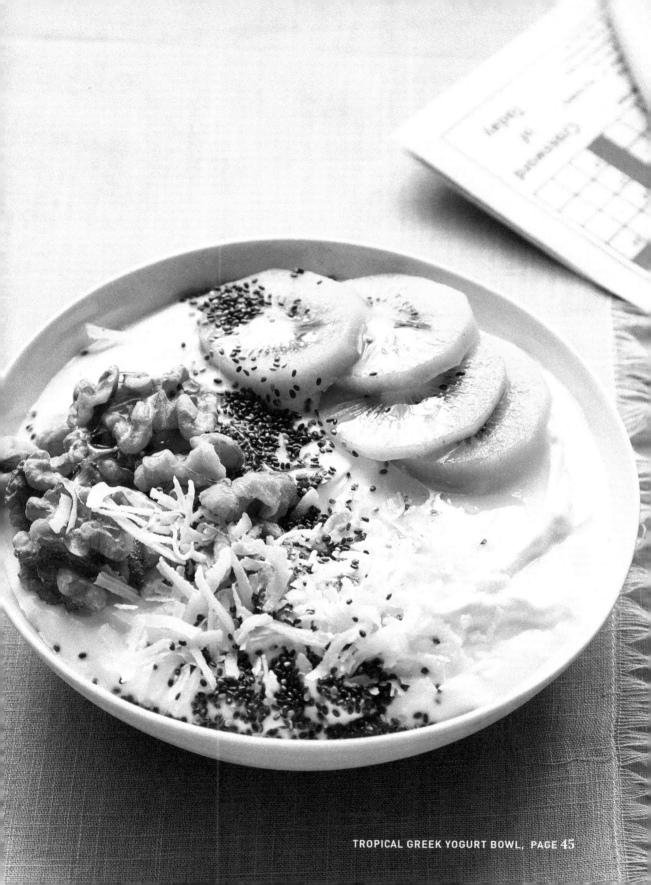

— CHAPTER THREE —

Breakfast

Berry Almond Smoothie

Carbs per serving: 19g

---

4 SERVINGS (7 OUNCES = 1 SERVING) | **PREP TIME:** 5 minutes

Smoothies are always a favorite because they're easy and require very little prep time. When I was pregnant, all I wanted to do was sleep, and getting those last few minutes mattered. On those sleepy mornings, I'd throw together a smoothie just before walking out the door and enjoy it on the way to class or another doctor's appointment. Use any berries you like for this recipe, or try a mix.

---

2 cups frozen berries of choice

1 cup plain low-fat Greek yogurt

1 cup unsweetened vanilla almond milk

½ cup natural almond butter

Put the berries, yogurt, almond milk, and almond butter into a blender and blend until smooth. If the smoothie is too thick, add more almond milk to thin.

COMPLETE THE MEAL: Pair this smoothie with Simple Grain-Free Biscuits (page 48), Coconut Pancakes (page 51), or Orange Muffins (page 49) for a proper portion of calories and carbs.

NUTRITIONAL INFORMATION: Calories: 277; Total Fat: 18g; Protein: 13g; Carbohydrates: 19g; Sugars: 11g; Fiber: 6g; Sodium: 140mg

Tropical Greek Yogurt Bowl

Carbs per serving: 23g

---

2 SERVINGS | **PREP TIME:** 5 minutes

This protein-packed breakfast can be made in minutes and will satisfy your morning hunger as well as your sweet tooth. This bowl tastes best when made fresh. If you are making breakfast only for yourself, consider cutting the recipe in half. If you are making it for the family, however, it is also easy to double.

1½ cups plain low-fat Greek yogurt

2 kiwis, peeled and sliced

2 tablespoons shredded unsweetened coconut flakes

2 tablespoons halved walnuts

1 tablespoon chia seeds

2 teaspoons honey, divided (optional)

1. Divide the yogurt between two small bowls.

2. Top each serving of yogurt with half of the kiwi slices, coconut flakes, walnuts, chia seeds, and honey (if using).

SUBSTITUTION TIP: Swap out the kiwi for ¼ cup berries or fresh pineapple, substitute flaxseed for chia seeds, or use toasted almonds instead of walnuts.

NUTRITIONAL INFORMATION: Calories: 260; Total Fat: 9g; Protein: 21g; Carbohydrates: 23g; Sugars: 14g; Fiber: 6g; Sodium: 83mg

Peanut Butter Power Oats

Carbs per serving: 27g

2 SERVINGS | **PREP TIME:** 5 minutes | **COOK TIME:** 5 minutes

A simple oatmeal recipe will keep you full without spiking your blood sugar. To make this recipe ahead of breakfast, divide the almond milk, oats, chia seeds, and peanut butter equally between two mason jars. Stir the ingredients, cover the jars, and place them in the refrigerator overnight. The next morning, enjoy the oats cold or heat them in the microwave for about 2 minutes. The covered jars can remain in the refrigerator for up to five days.

1½ cups unsweetened vanilla almond milk

¾ cup rolled oats

1 tablespoon chia seeds

2 tablespoons natural peanut butter

2 tablespoons walnut pieces, divided (optional)

¼ cup fresh berries, divided (optional)

1. In a small saucepan, bring the almond milk, oats, and chia seeds to a simmer.

2. Cover and cook, stirring frequently, until all of the milk is absorbed, and the chia seeds have gelled.

3. Add the peanut butter and stir until creamy.

4. Divide the oatmeal between two bowls. Top each serving with half of the walnuts and/or berries (if using).

INGREDIENT TIP: If gluten is a concern, look for a "gluten-free" certification on your ingredient labels to verify that proper measures have been taken to prevent cross-contamination in processing.

NUTRITIONAL INFORMATION: Calories: 261; Total Fat: 14g; Protein: 10g; Carbohydrates: 27g; Sugars: 1g; Fiber: 7g; Sodium: 131mg

Blueberry Coconut Breakfast Cookies

Carbs per serving: 28g

4 SERVINGS (3 COOKIES = 1 SERVING) | **PREP TIME:** 10 minutes | **COOK TIME:** 15 minutes

Who says you can't have cookies for breakfast? These cookies are a delightful alternative to a traditional breakfast, made possible by lower-carb sweeteners. Your family will love these, too—without having a clue how healthy they are.

4 tablespoons unsalted butter, at room temperature

2 medium bananas

4 large eggs

½ cup unsweetened applesauce

1 teaspoon vanilla extract

⅓ cup coconut flour

¼ teaspoon salt

1 cup fresh or frozen blueberries

1. Preheat the oven to 375°F.

2. In a medium bowl, mash the butter and bananas together with a fork until combined. The bananas can be a little chunky.

3. Add the eggs, applesauce, and vanilla to the bananas and mix well.

4. Stir in the coconut flour and salt.

5. Gently fold in the blueberries.

6. Drop about 2 tablespoons of dough on a baking sheet for each cookie and flatten it a bit with the back of a spoon. Bake for about 13 minutes, or until firm to the touch.

> **STORAGE TIP:** Store in a closed container in the refrigerator for up to 7 days.
>
> **COMPLETE THE MEAL:** Pair with 1 or 2 hardboiled eggs for added protein.

NUTRITIONAL INFORMATION: Calories: 305; Total Fat: 18g; Protein: 8g; Carbohydrates: 28g; Sugars: 15g; Fiber: 7g; Sodium: 222mg

Simple Grain-Free Biscuits

Carbs per serving: 9g

---

4 SERVINGS (1 BISCUIT = 1 SERVING) | **PREP TIME:** 10 minutes | **COOK TIME:** 15 minutes

You can still have biscuits for breakfast! Replacing all-purpose flour with almond flour adds healthy fat and protein while significantly reducing carbohydrates, and using Greek yogurt adds extra protein and probiotics. You don't need yeast, and you don't have to roll out the dough. Just drop it on a baking sheet, and in 15 minutes, you'll have low-carb biscuits that would be great with a drizzle of honey or some fruit.

---

2 tablespoons unsalted butter

Pinch salt

¼ cup plain low-fat Greek yogurt

1½ cups finely ground almond flour

1. Preheat the oven to 375°F.

2. In a medium bowl, microwave the butter just enough to soften, 15 to 20 seconds.

3. Add the salt and yogurt to the butter and mix well.

4. Add the almond flour and mix. The dough will be crumbly at first, so continue to stir and mash it with a fork until there are no lumps and the mixture comes together.

5. Drop ¼ cup of dough on a baking sheet for each biscuit. Using your clean hand, flatten each biscuit until it is 1 inch thick.

6. Bake for 13 to 15 minutes.

COMPLETE THE MEAL: Serve with a Berry Almond Smoothie (page 44), Loaded Avocado (page 52), or any of the egg dishes in this section.

NUTRITIONAL INFORMATION: Calories: 310; Total Fat: 28g; Protein: 10g; Carbohydrates: 9g; Sugars: 2g; Fiber: 5g; Sodium: 32mg

Orange Muffins

Carbs per serving: 16g

9 SERVINGS (1 MUFFIN = 1 SERVING) | **PREP TIME:** 15 minutes | **COOK TIME:** 15 minutes

Muffins are normally a food to avoid when managing GDM because they're often made with all-purpose flour and refined sugar. These muffins, however, contain low-carbohydrate replacements for the usual high-carb ingredients. The almond flour adds protein and reduces carbohydrates, and the fresh orange juice and honey add sweetness in the place of refined sugar.

2½ cups finely ground almond flour

¾ teaspoon ground cinnamon

½ teaspoon baking powder

½ teaspoon ground cardamom

¼ teaspoon salt

4 tablespoons avocado or coconut oil

2 large eggs

Grated zest and juice of 1 medium orange

1 tablespoon raw honey or 100% pure maple syrup

¼ teaspoon vanilla extract

1. Preheat the oven to 375°F.

2. In a large bowl, whisk together the almond flour, cinnamon, baking powder, cardamom, and salt. Set aside.

3. In a medium bowl, whisk together the oil, eggs, zest, juice, honey, and vanilla. Add this mixture to the dry ingredients, and stir until well combined.

4. In a nonstick muffin tin, fill each muffin cup until nearly full.

5. Bake for 15 minutes, or until the top center is firm.

COMPLETE THE MEAL: Feel free to have two servings of these yummy muffins for breakfast. You'll still be within your carb limit. Alternatively, consider pairing them with a side of eggs, such as the Brussels Sprouts and Egg Scramble (page 55).

NUTRITIONAL INFORMATION: Calories: 288; Total Fat: 23.6g; Protein: 8g; Carbohydrates: 16g; Sugars: 10g; Fiber: 4g; Sodium: 97mg

Crepe Cakes

Carbs per serving: 15g

4 SERVINGS (5 CAKES = 1 SERVING) | **PREP TIME:** 5 minutes | **COOK TIME:** 20 minutes

A hybrid of pancakes and crepes, these thin cakes are sweetened with banana instead of refined sugar. They also make a great dessert. For a special occasion, whip together 2 tablespoons coconut cream and ½ teaspoon 100% pure maple syrup, and add a small dollop to each serving.

Avocado oil cooking spray

4 ounces reduced-fat plain cream cheese, softened

2 medium bananas

4 large eggs

½ teaspoon vanilla extract

⅛ teaspoon salt

1. Heat a large skillet over low heat. Coat the cooking surface with cooking spray, and allow the pan to heat for another 2 to 3 minutes.

2. Meanwhile, in a medium bowl, mash the cream cheese and bananas together with a fork until combined. The bananas can be a little chunky.

3. Add the eggs, vanilla, and salt, and mix well.

4. For each cake, drop 2 tablespoons of the batter onto the warmed skillet and use the bottom of a large spoon or ladle to spread it thin. Let it cook for 7 to 9 minutes.

5. Flip the cake over and cook briefly, about 1 minute.

STORAGE TIP: Make a big batch of cakes and refrigerate them for up to 3 days. Reheat them in the microwave, as desired.

COMPLETE THE MEAL: Pair with Maple Sausage Frittata (page 57) or Huevos Rancheros Remix (page 54) for added calories, protein, and carbs.

NUTRITIONAL INFORMATION: Calories: 175; Total Fat: 9g; Protein: 9g; Carbohydrates: 15g; Sugars: 8g; Fiber: 2g; Sodium: 213mg

Coconut Pancakes

Carbs per serving: 10g

4 SERVINGS (2 PANCAKES = 1 SERVING) | **PREP TIME:** 5 minutes | **COOK TIME:** 15 to 20 minutes

Check out that carb count! Where else will you get two pancakes with just 10 carbs? Coconut flour is a great replacement for all-purpose flour when you want to cut carbs. It also makes these pancakes gluten-free, meaning you can make a big batch and warm them in the microwave when you're ready for more. They won't get tough like normal pancakes; instead, they'll taste like you just made them, every time.

½ cup coconut flour

1 teaspoon baking powder

½ teaspoon ground cinnamon

⅛ teaspoon salt

8 large eggs

⅓ cup unsweetened almond milk

2 tablespoons avocado or coconut oil

1 teaspoon vanilla extract

1. Heat a large skillet over medium-low heat.

2. In a large bowl, whisk together the flour, baking powder, cinnamon, and salt. Set aside.

3. In a medium bowl, whisk together the eggs, almond milk, oil, and vanilla. Pour the wet mixture into the dry ingredients and stir until combined.

4. Pour ⅓ cup of the batter onto the skillet for each pancake. Cook until bubbles appear on the surface of the pancake, about 7 minutes, then flip and cook for 1 minute more.

SUBSTITUTION TIP: The almond milk can be replaced with water without affecting the flavor. You can also swap the oil for butter for deeper flavor if dairy isn't a concern.

NUTRITIONAL INFORMATION: Calories: 270; Total Fat: 18g; Protein: 14g; Carbohydrates: 10g; Sugars: 2g; Fiber: 5g; Sodium: 325mg

Loaded Avocado

Carbs per serving: 11g

4 SERVINGS (½ AVOCADO + 2 EGGS = 1 SERVING) | **PREP TIME:** 5 minutes | **COOK TIME:** 5 minutes

Avocados—known for their healthy fat and yummy creaminess—are normally a topping in dishes, but they're the star in this flavorful and filling breakfast. The idea was inspired by a stuffed avocado dessert recipe made with almond butter and honey. This version is savory but still has a hint of sweetness from the red pepper spread. With a nice balance of protein, fat, and carbohydrates, it will set your blood sugar on the right track for the day.

Avocado oil cooking spray

8 large eggs

2 avocados

¼ cup Roasted Red Pepper Spread (page 142)

Fresh cilantro leaves, for garnish

Lime wedges, for garnish

1. Heat a large skillet over medium heat. When hot, coat the cooking surface with cooking spray and cook the eggs to your liking.

2. Meanwhile, cut the avocados in half lengthwise and remove the pits. Top each avocado half with 1 tablespoon of the red pepper spread.

3. For each portion, serve 2 eggs alongside 1 avocado half, and garnish with cilantro and a lime wedge.

INGREDIENT TIP: Since avocados brown quickly, cut only what you plan to serve immediately.

NUTRITIONAL INFORMATION: Calories: 283; Total Fat: 21g; Protein: 13g; Carbohydrates: 11g; Sugars: 3g; Fiber: 5g; Sodium: 280mg

Breakfast Tacos

Carbs per serving: 28g

4 SERVINGS | **PREP TIME:** 5 minutes | **COOK TIME:** 10 minutes

What I love about tacos is that you can eat all the ingredients separately, but when you make them into a taco, it's a game changer. You may be used to a more basic taqueria-style taco. But loading up on nutrients, like those found in bell peppers and spinach, is important for you and your baby—it's not just about counting carbs.

FOR THE TACO FILLING

Avocado oil cooking spray

1 medium green bell pepper, chopped

8 large eggs

¼ cup shredded sharp Cheddar cheese

4 (6-inch) whole-wheat tortillas

1 cup fresh spinach leaves

½ cup Pico de Gallo

Scallions, chopped, for garnish (optional)

Avocado slices, for garnish (optional)

FOR THE PICO DE GALLO

1 tomato, diced

½ large white onion, diced

2 tablespoons chopped fresh cilantro

½ jalapeño pepper, stemmed, seeded, and diced

1 tablespoon freshly squeezed lime juice

⅛ teaspoon salt

TO MAKE THE TACO FILLING

1. Heat a medium skillet over medium-low heat. When hot, coat the cooking surface with cooking spray and put the pepper in the skillet. Cook for 4 minutes.

2. Meanwhile, whisk the eggs in a medium bowl, then add the cheese and whisk to combine. Pour the eggs and cheese into the skillet with the green peppers and scramble until the eggs are fully cooked, about 5 minutes.

3. Microwave the tortillas very briefly, about 8 seconds.

4. For each serving, top a tortilla with one-quarter of the spinach, eggs, and pico de gallo. Garnish with scallions and avocado slices (if using).

TO MAKE THE PICO DE GALLO

In a medium bowl, combine the tomato, onion, cilantro, pepper, lime juice, and salt. Mix well and serve.

> **INGREDIENT TIP:** Pico de gallo has a bright, fresh flavor and is easy to make at home. Leftovers will keep in a covered container in the refrigerator for up to 2 days.

NUTRITIONAL INFORMATION: Calories: 276; Total Fat: 12g; Protein: 16g; Carbohydrates: 28g; Sugars: 8g; Fiber: 3g; Sodium: 562mg

Huevos Rancheros Remix

Carbs per serving: 18g

4 SERVINGS | **PREP TIME:** 5 minutes | **COOK TIME:** 10 minutes

Eggs are an amazing superfood, especially for pregnancy. They are very high in choline, which is a nutrient important for your baby's brain development. But eating plain eggs every day can get repetitive, and this recipe is a great way to liven them up.

1 cup low-sodium black beans, drained and rinsed

Avocado oil cooking spray

½ cup jarred salsa verde

8 large eggs

1 cup packaged or fresh Pico de Gallo (see page 53)

4 lime wedges

1. Pour the black beans and salsa verde into a small saucepan over low heat and cover. Cook until the beans are heated through, about 10 minutes.

2. Meanwhile, heat a small skillet over medium-low heat. When hot, coat the cooking surface with cooking spray, and fry or scramble the eggs to your liking.

3. For each portion, top 2 eggs with one-quarter of the black beans and pico de gallo. Finish each portion with a squeeze of lime.

INGREDIENT TIP: Save the remaining black beans to use in Southwest Salad (page 67) or Cauli-Flowing Sweet Potato (page 88) recipes.

COMPLETE THE MEAL: Pair with ½ cup berries or ½ piece of fruit to balance the protein in this dish with a proper portion of carbohydrates.

NUTRITIONAL INFORMATION: Calories: 210; Total Fat: 9.4g; Protein: 15g; Carbohydrates: 18g; Sugars: 4g; Fiber: 5g; Sodium: 439mg

Brussels Sprouts and Egg Scramble

Carbs per serving: 10g

---

4 SERVINGS | **PREP TIME:** 5 minutes | **COOK TIME:** 20 minutes

---

This seemingly unconventional breakfast idea is full of nutrients. For variation, try this with another leafy green vegetable, like spinach or chard. Sauté the greens with the bacon in step 2 and skip step 4. You may also want to experiment with different cheeses—goat cheese or blue cheese would complement any of the green vegetables.

Avocado oil cooking spray

4 slices low-sodium turkey bacon

20 Brussels sprouts, halved lengthwise

8 large eggs

¼ cup crumbled feta, for garnish

1. Heat a large skillet over medium heat. When hot, coat the cooking surface with cooking spray and cook the bacon to your liking.

2. Carefully remove the bacon from the pan and set it on a plate lined with a paper towel to drain and cool.

3. Place the Brussels sprouts in the skillet cut-side down, and cook for 3 minutes.

4. Reduce the heat to medium-low. Flip the Brussels sprouts, move them to one side of the skillet, and cover. Cook for another 3 minutes.

5. Uncover. Cook the eggs to over-medium alongside the Brussels sprouts, or to your liking.

6. Crumble the bacon once it has cooled.

7. Divide the Brussels sprouts into 4 portions and top each portion with one-quarter of the crumbled bacon and 2 eggs. Add 1 tablespoon of feta to each portion.

INGREDIENT TIP: Use the remaining turkey bacon for Chicken Tender and Brussels Sprout Cobb Salad (page 71).

COMPLETE THE MEAL: Pair this dish with a small piece of fruit, 1 cup berries, Simple Grain-Free Biscuits (page 48), or Orange Muffins (page 49) to get adequate carbs and calories from your morning meal.

NUTRITIONAL INFORMATION: Calories: 253; Total Fat: 15g; Protein: 21g; Carbohydrates: 10g; Sugars: 4g; Fiber: 4g; Sodium: 343mg

Sausage, Sweet Potato, and Kale Hash

Carbs per serving: 32g

4 SERVINGS | **PREP TIME:** 10 minutes | **COOK TIME:** 15 minutes

Outside of eggs and meats, many typical breakfast foods are high carb, so it's important to reimagine what breakfast can be. This dish keeps the breakfast feel with eggs and sausage but strays from tradition with kale and sweet potatoes. A squeeze of lemon at the end brings the flavors together.

Avocado oil cooking spray

1⅓ cups peeled and diced sweet potatoes

8 cups roughly chopped kale, stemmed and loosely packed (about 2 bunches)

4 links chicken or turkey breakfast sausage

4 large eggs

4 lemon wedges

1. Heat a large skillet over medium heat. When hot, coat the cooking surface with cooking spray. Cook the sweet potatoes for 4 minutes, stirring once halfway through.

2. Reduce the heat to medium-low and move the potatoes to one side of the skillet. Arrange the kale and sausage in a single layer. Cover and cook for 3 minutes.

3. Stir the vegetables and sausage together, then push them to one side of the skillet to create space for the eggs. Add the eggs and cook them to your liking. Cover the skillet and cook for 3 minutes.

4. Divide the sausage and vegetables into four equal portions and top with an egg and a squeeze of lemon.

> **OPTION:** If you need to reduce the carb count, cut the amount of sweet potatoes in half.

NUTRITIONAL INFORMATION: Calories: 234; Total Fat: 8g; Protein: 12g; Carbohydrates: 32g; Sugars: 6g; Fiber: 5g; Sodium: 270mg

Maple Sausage Frittata

Carbs per serving: 10g

4 SERVINGS | **PREP TIME:** 10 minutes | **COOK TIME:** 15 minutes

Experimenting with new flavors is a great way to keep mealtimes exciting. Frittatas originated in Italy, and this one is sweet, savory, and earthy, making it somewhat reminiscent of Asian cuisine. Because this frittata uses almond milk, it can be reheated without making the eggs rubbery, so this is a great breakfast to make ahead for weekday mornings.

Avocado oil cooking spray

1 cup roughly chopped portobello mushrooms

1 medium green bell pepper, diced

1 medium red bell pepper, diced

8 large eggs

¾ cup half-and-half

¼ cup unsweetened almond milk

6 links maple-flavored chicken or turkey breakfast sausage, cut into ¼-inch pieces

1. Preheat the oven to 375°F.

2. Heat a large, oven-safe skillet over medium-low heat. When hot, coat the cooking surface with cooking spray.

3. Heat the mushrooms, green bell pepper, and red bell pepper in the skillet. Cook for 5 minutes.

4. Meanwhile, in a medium bowl, whisk the eggs, half-and-half, and almond milk.

5. Add the sausage to the skillet and cook for 2 minutes.

6. Pour the egg mixture into the skillet, then transfer the skillet from the stove to the oven, and bake for 15 minutes, or until the middle is firm and spongy.

INGREDIENT TIP: Buying an 8-ounce package of presliced portobello mushrooms for this recipe and chopping them into quarters will save time.

COMPLETE THE MEAL: Pair with Crepe Cakes (page 50), Orange Muffins (page 49), or a small whole fruit to get an adequate carb count.

NUTRITIONAL INFORMATION: Calories: 280; Total Fat: 17g; Protein: 21g; Carbohydrates: 10g; Sugars: 7g; Fiber: 2g; Sodium: 446mg

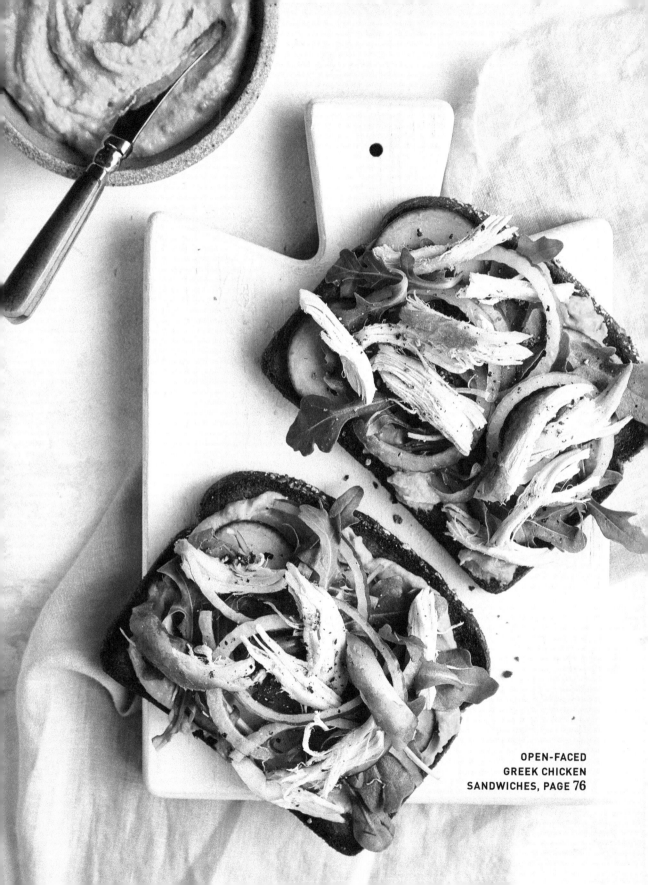

OPEN-FACED
GREEK CHICKEN
SANDWICHES, PAGE 76

Soups, Salads, Sandwiches

Cauliflower Leek Soup

Carbs per serving: 24g

---

2 SERVINGS (¾ CUP = 1 SERVING) | **PREP TIME:** 10 minutes | **COOK TIME:** 20 minutes

---

Leeks are a great way to add flavor to a dish. When using leeks, be sure to thoroughly clean them. Cut off the root end at the bottom and the tops where the leaves begin to turn green. Discard the tough outer leaves. Cut the leeks in half lengthwise and rinse them under cold running water, feathering water through the leaves to dislodge any soil, then prepare as directed (for this recipe, chop them into ½-inch pieces).

Avocado oil cooking spray

2½ cups chopped leeks (2 to 3 leeks)

2½ cups cauliflower florets

1 garlic clove, peeled

⅓ cup low-sodium vegetable broth

½ cup half-and-half

¼ teaspoon salt

¼ teaspoon freshly ground black pepper

1. Heat a large stockpot over medium-low heat. When hot, coat the cooking surface with cooking spray. Put the leeks and cauliflower into the pot.

2. Increase the heat to medium and cover the pan. Cook for 10 minutes, stirring halfway through.

3. Add the garlic and cook for 5 minutes.

4. Add the broth and deglaze the pan, stirring to scrape up the browned bits from the bottom.

5. Transfer the broth and vegetables to a food processor or blender and add the half-and-half, salt, and pepper. Blend well.

INGREDIENT TIP: Save any leftover cauliflower for Cauli-Flowing Sweet Potato (page 88) or Easy Everyday Veggie Bowl (page 84).

COMPLETE THE MEAL: For added protein, pair this soup with a meat, fish, or poultry dish, such as Coconut Lime Chicken (page 108) or Lemon Pepper Salmon (page 132).

NUTRITIONAL INFORMATION: Calories: 173; Total Fat: 7g; Protein: 6g; Carbohydrates: 24g; Sugars: 8g; Fiber: 5g; Sodium: 487mg

Slow Cooker Chicken and Vegetable Soup

Carbs per serving: 25g

---

4 SERVINGS (3½ CUPS = 1 SERVING) | **PREP TIME:** 10 minutes | **COOK TIME:** 4 hours

---

A slow-cooked meal will always be a winner. My mom made slow-cooked meals so often that I got tired of seeing the slow cooker on the kitchen counter. As a busy adult, I now know that this dependable appliance can be a lifesaver. You can throw everything in before you leave for work and have a no-hassle dinner ready by the time you get home.

---

1 medium potato, peeled and chopped into 1-inch pieces

3 celery stalks, chopped into 1-inch pieces

2 cups chopped baby carrots

1 cup chopped white onion

2 cups chopped green beans

2 cups low-sodium chicken broth

2 tablespoons tomato paste

2 tablespoons Italian seasoning

1 pound boneless, skinless chicken breasts, chopped

Freshly ground black pepper

1. Put the potato, celery, carrots, onion, green beans, broth, tomato paste, Italian seasoning, and chicken into a slow cooker and cook on high for 4 hours.

2. Season with freshly ground black pepper.

OPTION: Top individual servings with 1 tablespoon shredded or grated Parmesan cheese.

SUBSTITUTION TIP: This recipe can be adapted to vegetables you have on hand or to your personal preferences. Make sure the vegetables you use are nonstarchy, such as bell peppers, cauliflower, eggplant, leafy greens, mushrooms, or zucchini.

NUTRITIONAL INFORMATION: Calories: 232; Total Fat: 3g; Protein: 30g; Carbohydrates: 25g; Sugars: 7g; Fiber: 6g; Sodium: 180mg

Cheeseburger Soup

Carbs per serving: 9g

4 SERVINGS (1¾ CUPS = 1 SERVING) | **PREP TIME:** 5 minutes | **COOK TIME:** 25 minutes

This soup is everything you love about a cheeseburger and so deep in flavor you won't even miss the bun. It can be hard to adjust to eating less bread while managing gestational diabetes, but turning a favorite recipe into a soup is a great way to reduce the carbs while keeping your meals filling and satisfying.

Avocado oil cooking spray

½ cup diced white onion

½ cup diced celery

½ cup sliced
portobello mushrooms

1 pound 93% lean
ground beef

1 (15-ounce) can no-salt-
added diced tomatoes

2 cups low-sodium
beef broth

⅓ cup half-and-half

¾ cup shredded sharp
Cheddar cheese

1. Heat a large stockpot over medium-low heat. When hot, coat the cooking surface with cooking spray. Put the onion, celery, and mushrooms into the pot. Cook for 7 minutes, stirring occasionally.

2. Add the ground beef and cook for 5 minutes, stirring and breaking apart as needed.

3. Add the diced tomatoes with their juices and the broth. Increase the heat to medium-high and simmer for 10 minutes.

4. Remove the pot from the heat and stir in the half-and-half.

5. Serve topped with the cheese.

SUBSTITUTION TIP: You can substitute 93% lean ground turkey for the ground beef and low-sodium chicken broth for the beef broth, if desired.

COMPLETE THE MEAL: Serve this soup with a side of 1 to 2 cups steamed, grilled, or raw vegetables of your choice or a vegetable dish, such as Italian Zucchini Boats (page 93), to balance the fat and protein with adequate carbohydrates.

NUTRITIONAL INFORMATION: Calories: 330; Total Fat: 18g; Protein: 33g; Carbohydrates: 9g; Sugars: 5g; Fiber: 2g; Sodium: 321mg

Taco Soup

Carbs per serving: 23g

4 SERVINGS (2½ CUPS = 1 SERVING) | **PREP TIME:** 5 minutes | **COOK TIME:** 20 minutes

This easy soup is full of flavor. Replacing packaged taco seasoning with a homemade mix of spices—cumin, chili powder, garlic powder—significantly lowers the sodium in this recipe. Feel free to experiment with seasoning proportions to suit your personal taste.

Avocado oil cooking spray

1 medium red bell pepper, chopped

½ cup chopped yellow onion

1 pound 93% lean ground beef

1 teaspoon ground cumin

½ teaspoon salt

½ teaspoon chili powder

½ teaspoon garlic powder

2 cups low-sodium beef broth

1 (15-ounce) can no-salt-added diced tomatoes

1½ cups frozen corn

⅓ cup half-and-half

1. Heat a large stockpot over medium-low heat. When hot, coat the cooking surface with cooking spray. Put the pepper and onion in the pan and cook for 5 minutes.

2. Add the ground beef, cumin, salt, chili powder, and garlic powder. Cook for 5 to 7 minutes, stirring and breaking apart the beef as needed.

3. Add the broth, diced tomatoes with their juices, and corn. Increase the heat to medium-high and simmer for 10 minutes.

4. Remove from the heat and stir in the half-and-half.

SUBSTITUTION TIP: You can substitute 93% lean ground turkey for the ground beef and low-sodium chicken broth for the beef broth, if desired.

COMPLETE THE MEAL: To get an adequate amount of carbs, serve this soup with 1 cup steamed, grilled, or raw vegetables.

NUTRITIONAL INFORMATION: Calories: 320; Total Fat: 12g; Protein: 30g; Carbohydrates: 23g; Sugars: 7g; Fiber: 4g; Sodium: 456mg

Low-Carb Ramen with Pork Loin

Carbs per serving: 16g

---

4 SERVINGS (2 CUPS = 1 SERVING) | **PREP TIME:** 5 minutes | **COOK TIME:** 20 minutes

---

Do you know why takeout is so popular? Not only is it delicious, but it often requires a lot of prep work, and to do that at home for just one meal isn't ideal. The problem with takeout, however, is that it's hard to assess how much sodium and carbohydrates might be in it. This recipe lets you enjoy a takeout favorite and control the ingredients.

---

1 tablespoon sesame oil

2 cups sliced portobello or shiitake mushrooms

1 teaspoon garlic powder

½ teaspoon ground ginger

6 cups low-sodium beef broth

1 cup water

2 teaspoons low-sodium soy sauce

4 teaspoons rice vinegar

½ teaspoon fish sauce

5 sheets snack-size nori

2 cups packaged carrot noodles or preferred vegetable noodles

1 pound Roasted Pork Loin (page 114)

¼ cup chopped scallions (optional)

1. Heat a large stockpot over medium heat. When hot, pour in the sesame oil, then add the mushrooms, garlic powder, and ginger. Cook for 5 minutes, stirring occasionally.

2. Pour in the broth and water, then add the soy sauce, rice vinegar, and fish sauce. Increase the heat to high and bring the broth to a boil.

3. Chop the nori into ¼-inch strips.

4. When the soup begins to boil, add the noodles and nori, and cook for 3 minutes.

5. Cut the pork loin into 8 even slices.

6. Divide the soup between 4 bowls, and top each portion with 2 slices of pork loin and 1 tablespoon of chopped scallions (if using).

OPTION: Add a sliced medium-boiled egg to the top of each serving.

MAKE-AHEAD TIP: Make Roasted Pork Loin (page 114) (without the vegetables) when you have a little bit of extra time. You can keep the cooked pork loin in the refrigerator in a covered container for 3 to 4 days.

COMPLETE THE MEAL: Enjoy this soup with a side of vegetables, such as 1 cup steamed broccoli or 1 cup shelled edamame.

NUTRITIONAL INFORMATION: Calories: 362; Total Fat: 17g; Protein: 38g; Carbohydrates: 16g; Sugars: 7g; Fiber: 5g; Sodium: 396mg

Summer Salad

Carbs per serving: 22g

4 SERVINGS | **PREP TIME:** 5 minutes

This simple salad is perfect for a warm summer afternoon. The peaches give it a touch of natural sweetness, the onion gives it bite, the walnuts add a perfect crunch, and the feta lends a creamy finish. Even though peaches contain sugar, you can still enjoy them in reasonable amounts.

FOR THE SALAD

8 cups mixed greens or preferred lettuce, loosely packed

4 cups arugula, loosely packed

2 peaches, sliced

½ cup thinly sliced red onion

½ cup chopped walnuts or pecans

½ cup crumbled feta

FOR THE DRESSING

4 teaspoons extra-virgin olive oil

4 teaspoons honey

TO MAKE THE SALAD

1. Combine the mixed greens, arugula, peaches, red onion, walnuts, and feta in a large bowl. Divide the salad into four portions.

2. Drizzle the dressing over each individual serving of salad.

TO MAKE THE DRESSING

In a small bowl, whisk together the olive oil and honey.

LEFTOVER TIP: To prevent the salad from getting soggy, add dressing only to the portion you are ready to eat. Store leftover salad and dressing separately in the refrigerator to save for the next day.

COMPLETE THE MEAL: Pair this salad with a protein dish, such as Roasted Pork Loin (page 114) or Peppered Chicken with Balsamic Kale (page 102).

NUTRITIONAL INFORMATION: Calories: 263; Total Fat: 18g; Protein: 8g; Carbohydrates: 22g; Sugars: 16g; Fiber: 5g; Sodium: 222mg

Greek Chickpea Salad

Carbs per serving: 23g

4 SERVINGS | **PREP TIME:** 5 minutes

This is a classic salad that can be eaten alone or as a satisfying side dish. The water content in the cucumber and tomato helps make it filling, but you're also getting protein from the chickpeas and the Greek yogurt dressing. The best way to create larger portions for this salad is to increase the cucumbers and tomatoes, which won't significantly raise the carbohydrates or sodium.

2 cups diced cucumber

2 cups diced tomatoes

1½ cups canned low-sodium chickpeas, drained and rinsed

½ cup sliced red onion

¼ cup crumbled feta

8 pitted green olives, drained, rinsed, and halved

¾ cup Creamy Dill Dressing (page 140)

In a large bowl, combine the cucumber, tomatoes, chickpeas, red onion, feta, and olives. Add the dressing and stir.

COMPLETE THE MEAL: For added protein, consider pairing this salad with 4 ounces grilled chicken or fish and additional vegetables dipped in any remaining dill dressing or ¼ cup hummus.

NUTRITIONAL INFORMATION: Calories: 190; Total Fat: 7g; Protein: 10g; Carbohydrates: 22g; Sugars: 8g; Fiber: 6g; Sodium: 477mg

Southwest Salad

Carbs per serving: 30g

4 SERVINGS | **PREP TIME:** 5 minutes | **COOK TIME:** 10 minutes

Southwest salads can often have too many carbs—from corn, beans, and tortilla strips, if included. This recipe allows you to enjoy this classic salad while accommodating your nutritional needs by reducing the beans and adding other ingredients with southwestern flavors, like sweet potatoes and avocado dressing.

1 cup cubed frozen or fresh sweet potato

4 cups frozen or fresh broccoli florets

8 cups mixed greens or preferred lettuce, loosely packed

1 cup canned low-sodium black beans, drained and rinsed

1 cup Creamy Avocado Dressing (page 139)

1. Prepare the sweet potatoes and broccoli according to the package instructions if frozen.

2. In a large bowl, combine the sweet potatoes, broccoli, greens, black beans, and avocado dressing. Toss well.

INGREDIENT TIP: Save the remaining black beans for Huevos Rancheros Remix (page 54) or Cauli-Flowing Sweet Potato (page 88).

NUTRITIONAL INFORMATION: Calories: 195; Total Fat: 8g; Protein: 10g; Carbohydrates: 30g; Sugars: 3g; Fiber: 6g; Sodium: 53mg

Kidney Bean Salad

Carbs per serving: 36g

4 SERVINGS | **PREP TIME:** 10 minutes

This is a great salad to pair with white fish, chicken, or turkey. The bulk of the carbs come from the beans and the corn. Kidney beans have good protein and fiber, so reduce the corn if you'd like to cut the carbs a bit. Kidney beans are also high in iron, which is necessary for fetal brain development, and magnesium, which can help ease nausea.

3 cups diced cucumber

1 (15-ounce) can low-sodium dark red kidney beans, drained and rinsed

2 avocados, diced

1½ cups diced tomatoes

1 cup cooked corn

¾ cup sliced red onion

1 tablespoon extra-virgin olive oil

1 tablespoon apple cider vinegar

In a large bowl, combine the cucumber, kidney beans, avocados, tomatoes, corn, onion, olive oil, and vinegar.

COMPLETE THE MEAL: Serve as a side dish with Sofrito Beef Tips (page 122), Coconut Lime Chicken (page 108), or Cheeseburger and Cauliflower Wraps (page 118).

NUTRITIONAL INFORMATION: Calories: 316; Total Fat: 16g; Protein: 10g; Carbohydrates: 36g; Sugars: 7g; Fiber: 14g; Sodium: 116mg

Chicken, Spinach, and Berry Salad

Carbs per serving: 13g

4 SERVINGS | **PREP TIME:** 5 minutes

When you find ingredients that sing together, your senses sing with them. That's what you can expect with this salad. This tasty meal is packed with healthy proteins, fats, and carbs. If you want to add more healthy carbs, try the salad with ½ cup chickpeas.

FOR THE SALAD

8 cups baby spinach

2 cups shredded rotisserie chicken

½ cup sliced strawberries or other berries

½ cup sliced almonds

1 avocado, sliced

¼ cup crumbled feta (optional)

FOR THE DRESSING

2 tablespoons extra-virgin olive oil

2 teaspoons honey

2 teaspoons balsamic vinegar

TO MAKE THE SALAD

1. In a large bowl, combine the spinach, chicken, strawberries, and almonds.

2. Pour the dressing over the salad and lightly toss.

3. Divide into four equal portions and top each with sliced avocado and 1 tablespoon of crumbled feta (if using).

TO MAKE THE DRESSING

In a small bowl, whisk together the olive oil, honey, and balsamic vinegar.

COMPLETE THE MEAL: To achieve the right balance of carbohydrates, pair this salad with a vegetarian side dish, such as Chickpea Coconut Curry (page 95) or an additional 1 cup strawberries per serving.

NUTRITIONAL INFORMATION: Calories: 339; Total F... 25g; Carbohydrates: 13g; Sugars: 6g; Fiber: 6g; Sodium...

Chicken, Cantaloupe, Kale, and Almond Salad

Carbs per serving: 24g

---

3 SERVINGS | **PREP TIME:** 10 minutes

On the days that you want to go lighter, this is a perfect meal to throw together quickly—with no cooking. Since cantaloupe is in season during the summer, this is a great salad to eat on hot days. If don't want the heartiness or texture of the kale, try baby kale (it's more tender) or spinach.

FOR THE SALAD

4 cups chopped kale, packed

1½ cups diced cantaloupe

1½ cups shredded rotisserie chicken

½ cup sliced almonds

¼ cup crumbled feta

FOR THE DRESSING

2 teaspoons honey

**2 tablespoons extra-
v̶i̶̶ ̶ ̶ ̶o̶i̶l̶**

**2 teasp̶
cider vinega̶̶̶̶ly
squeezed lemon**

TO MAKE THE SALAD

1. Divide the kale into three portions. Layer ⅓ of the cantaloupe, chicken, almonds, and feta on each portion.

2. Drizzle some of the dressing over each portion of salad. Serve immediately.

TO MAKE THE DRESSING

In a small bowl, whisk together the honey, olive oil, and vinegar.

COMPLETE THE MEAL: Have an additional 1 cup cubed cantaloupe with each serving to reach proper carb count.

NUTRITIONAL INFORMATION: Calories: 396; Total Fat: 22g; Protein: 27g; Carbohydrates: 24g; Sugars: 12g; Fiber: 4g; Sodium: 236mg

Chicken Tender and Brussels Sprout Cobb Salad

Carbs per serving: 37g

4 SERVINGS | **PREP TIME:** 10 minutes | **COOK TIME:** 30 minutes

Sweet, savory, and tangy, this salad hits all the right notes and is a great meal to prep ahead and have for lunch throughout the week. Because all of the ingredients can be eaten cold, it makes a great grab-and-go option. If you prefer, you can store the meats separately and warm them before adding them to the salad.

FOR THE SALAD

8 (2-ounce) chicken tenders

2 slices turkey bacon

2 (9-ounce) packages shaved Brussels sprouts

2 hardboiled eggs, chopped

½ cup unsweetened dried cranberries

FOR THE DRESSING

3 tablespoons honey mustard

3 tablespoons extra-virgin olive oil

½ tablespoon freshly squeezed lemon juice

TO MAKE THE SALAD

1. Preheat the oven to 425°F.

2. Lightly coat the chicken tenders with cooking spray, then place them on a baking sheet and bake for 15 to 18 minutes.

3. Meanwhile, heat a large skillet over medium-low heat. When hot, fry the bacon for 5 to 7 minutes until crispy. When the bacon is done, carefully remove it from the pan, and set it on a plate lined with a paper towel to drain and cool. Crumble when cool enough to handle.

4. Cut the chicken tenders into even pieces. Divide the Brussels sprouts into four equal portions. Top each portion with one-quarter of the chopped eggs and crumbled bacon and 2 sliced chicken tenders.

5. Drizzle an equal portion of dressing over each serving.

TO MAKE THE DRESSING

In a small bowl, whisk together the mustard, olive oil, and lemon juice.

LEFTOVER TIP: Use the remaining turkey bacon in Brussels Sprouts and Egg Scramble (page 55).

NUTRITIONAL INFORMATION: Calories: 468; Total Fat: 20g; Protein: 35g; Carbohydrates: 37g; Sugars: 14g; Fiber: 10g; Sodium: 242mg

Sofrito Steak Salad

Carbs per serving: 18g

4 SERVINGS | **PREP TIME:** 10 minutes | **COOK TIME:** 15 minutes

Recaíto is a Puerto Rican base ingredient used in *sofrito* to flavor meat, beans, soups, and stews. It is made with onion, garlic, assorted peppers, and lots of cilantro. You can find *recaíto* in the Latin foods section of your supermarket. This salad is perfect for GDM because it's naturally low-carb and full of nutrient-rich ingredients.

4 ounces *recaíto* cooking base

2 (4-ounce) flank steaks

8 cups fresh spinach, loosely packed

½ cup sliced red onion

2 cups diced tomato

2 avocados, diced

2 cups diced cucumber

⅓ cup crumbled feta

1. Heat a large skillet over medium-low heat. When hot, pour in the *recaíto* cooking base, add the steaks, and cover. Cook for 8 to 12 minutes.

2. Meanwhile, divide the spinach into four portions. Top each portion with one-quarter of the onion, tomato, avocados, and cucumber.

3. Remove the steak from the skillet, and let it rest for about 2 minutes before slicing. Place one-quarter of the steak and feta on top of each portion.

OPTION: Use the *recaíto* cooking base from the skillet as a dressing, or drizzle 1 tablespoon extra-virgin olive oil or 1 tablespoon balsamic or raspberry vinaigrette on top of each portion.

NUTRITIONAL INFORMATION: Calories: 344; Total Fat: 18g; Protein: 25g; Carbohydrates: 18g; Sugars: 6g; Fiber: 8g; Sodium: 382mg

Open-Faced Egg Salad Sandwiches

Carbs per serving: 23g

---

4 SERVINGS (1 SLICE OF BREAD WITH TOPPINGS = 1 SERVING) | **PREP TIME:** 10 minutes

---

Egg salad sandwiches are great for three reasons: (1) they're easy to make, (2) they're filling, and (3) eggs are a superfood with amazing benefits for both you and your baby. To get the full benefits of eggs, you have to eat the white and the yolk, as most of the nutrients are packed into the yolk. Choline, DHA, and folate are all found in eggs and are vital to your baby's brain and nervous system development.

---

8 large hardboiled eggs

3 tablespoons plain low-fat Greek yogurt

1 tablespoon mustard

½ teaspoon freshly ground black pepper

1 teaspoon chopped fresh chives

4 slices 100% whole-wheat bread

2 cups fresh spinach, loosely packed

1. Peel the eggs and cut them in half.

2. In a large bowl, mash the eggs with a fork, leaving chunks.

3. Add the yogurt, mustard, pepper, and chives, and mix.

4. For each portion, layer 1 slice of bread with one-quarter of the egg salad and spinach.

COMPLETE THE MEAL: Have a small piece of fruit or ½ cup veggie sticks dipped in ¼ cup hummus for a balanced meal.

NUTRITIONAL INFORMATION: Calories: 277; Total Fat: 12g; Protein: 20g; Carbohydrates: 23g; Sugars: 3g; Fiber: 3g; Sodium: 364mg

Chicken Salad Sandwiches

Carbs per serving: 24g

4 SERVINGS | **PREP TIME:** 10 minutes | **COOK TIME:** 10 minutes, plus 5 minutes to cool

Normally, chicken salad is made with mayonnaise, but replacing it with plain low-fat Greek yogurt reduces the fat and adds great benefits, like probiotics for your gut, extra protein, vitamin B_{12}, and more. This recipe is just as delicious as traditional chicken salad, and it's quick and easy to make.

Avocado oil cooking spray

2 (4-ounce) boneless, skinless chicken breasts

⅛ teaspoon freshly ground black pepper

1½ tablespoons plain low-fat Greek yogurt

¼ cup halved purple seedless grapes

¼ cup chopped pecans

2 tablespoons chopped celery

4 sandwich thins, 100% whole-wheat

1. Heat a small skillet over medium-low heat. When hot, coat the cooking surface with cooking spray.

2. Season the chicken with the pepper. Place the chicken in the skillet and cook for 6 minutes. Flip and cook for 3 to 5 minutes more, or until cooked through.

3. Remove the chicken from the skillet and let cool for 5 minutes.

4. Chop or shred the chicken.

5. Combine the chicken, yogurt, grapes, pecans, and celery.

6. Cut the sandwich thins in half, so there is a top and bottom.

7. Divide the chicken salad into four equal portions, spoon one portion on each of the bottom halves of the sandwich thins, and cover with the top halves.

INGREDIENT TIP: Save time by buying a cooked rotisserie chicken instead of cooking the chicken breasts, or use 1 (8-ounce) can of chunk chicken breast, drained.

REPURPOSE: Double the recipe (minus the sandwich thins), and save half for a quick Chicken Salad Salad (page 100).

NUTRITIONAL INFORMATION: Calories: 250; Total Fat: 8g; Protein: 23g; Carbohydrates: 24g; Sugars: 4g; Fiber: 6g; Sodium: 209mg

Caesar Chicken Sandwiches

Carbs per serving: 25g

4 SERVINGS | **PREP TIME:** 5 minutes

Have you ever looked at the nutrition facts on salad dressings? They often have added sugars. Store-bought Caesar dressing can also have excess sodium, but homemade dressing can easily achieve the same flavor and texture without the added salt. Give it a try.

FOR THE DRESSING

4 tablespoons plain low-fat Greek yogurt

4 teaspoons Dijon mustard

4 teaspoons freshly squeezed lemon juice

4 teaspoons shredded Parmesan cheese

¼ teaspoon freshly ground black pepper

⅛ teaspoon garlic powder

FOR THE SANDWICHES

2 cups shredded rotisserie chicken

1½ cups chopped romaine lettuce

12 cherry tomatoes, halved

4 sandwich thins, 100% whole-wheat

¼ cup thinly sliced red onion (optional)

TO MAKE THE DRESSING

In a small bowl, whisk together the yogurt, mustard, lemon juice, Parmesan cheese, black pepper, and garlic powder.

TO MAKE THE SANDWICHES

1. In a large bowl, combine the chicken, lettuce, and tomatoes. Add the dressing and stir until evenly coated. Divide the filling into four equal portions.

2. Slice the sandwich thins so there is a top and bottom half for each. Put one portion of filling on each of the bottom halves and cover with the top halves.

INGREDIENT TIP: Save the remaining rotisserie chicken for Open-Faced Greek Chicken Sandwiches (page 76), Chicken Salad Salad (page 100), or Chicken, Spinach, and Berry Salad (page 69).

NUTRITIONAL INFORMATION: Calories: 242; Total Fat: 5g; Protein: 28g; Carbohydrates: 25g; Sugars: 4g; Fiber: 8g; Sodium: 359mg

Open-Faced Greek Chicken Sandwiches

Carbs per serving: 25g

---

3 SERVINGS (1 SLICE OF BREAD, TOPPED = 1 SERVING) | **PREP TIME:** 10 minutes

---

The great thing about new ways of eating is that they introduce you to new flavor combinations that you might not have considered before. The texture of toasted bread with creamy hummus, crisp cucumber and onion slices, fresh greens, and the deep flavor of rotisserie chicken create a symphony of Greek-inspired flavors in your mouth. If you have it on hand, a sprinkle of fresh oregano will put these sandwiches over the top.

---

3 tablespoons red pepper hummus

3 slices 100% whole-wheat bread, toasted

¾ cup cucumber slices

3 cups arugula or baby kale

¼ cup sliced red onion

1 cup shredded rotisserie chicken

Oregano, for garnish (optional)

1. Spread 1 tablespoon of hummus on each slice of toasted bread.

2. Layer one-third of the cucumber, arugula, onion, and chicken on each slice of bread. Garnish with oregano (if using).

> **INGREDIENT TIP:** Save the remaining chicken for Open-Faced Chicken and Onion Grilled Cheese (page 77) or Chicken, Spinach, and Berry Salad (page 69).

NUTRITIONAL INFORMATION: Calories: 228; Total Fat: 6g; Protein: 23g; Carbohydrates: 25g; Sugars: 4g; Fiber: 4g; Sodium: 331mg

Open-Faced Chicken and Onion Grilled Cheese

Carbs per serving: 23g

---

4 SERVINGS (1 SLICE OF BREAD WITH TOPPINGS = 1 SERVING)
PREP TIME: 10 minutes | **COOK TIME:** 15 minutes

Taking the traditional grilled cheese up a notch, this sandwich gives you more flavor bang for your buck. A normal grilled cheese doesn't provide much nutrition or enough flavor to get excited about. Adding grilled onions, rotisserie chicken, and vitamin-rich spinach makes for a fun, nutritious twist on a classic.

---

1 small yellow onion

Avocado oil cooking spray

2 cups shredded rotisserie chicken

1½ tablespoons unsalted butter

4 slices 100% whole-wheat bread

3 slices provolone or Swiss cheese

2 cups fresh spinach

1. Cut the onion into ½-inch rounds. Leave them intact; do not separate.

2. Heat a medium or large skillet over medium-low heat. When hot, coat the cooking surface with cooking spray. Place the onions in the skillet. Cover and cook for 7 to 10 minutes, or until the onions are translucent. Remove from the skillet.

3. Meanwhile, shred the chicken, and butter one side of each slice of bread. Tear each slice of cheese into 3 strips.

4. Place 2 or 3 strips of cheese on the nonbuttered side of each piece of bread, then place the buttered side down on the skillet.

5. Layer one-quarter of the onion, spinach, and shredded chicken on top of each slice of bread.

6. Toast for 2 to 3 minutes over medium-low heat.

INGREDIENT TIP: Save leftover shredded rotisserie chicken for any of the chicken salad or sandwich recipes.

COMPLETE THE MEAL: Pair with fruit or vegetables, such as ¼ cup grapes, ½ pear, or ½ cup veggie sticks dipped in ¼ cup hummus, for a balanced meal.

NUTRITIONAL INFORMATION: Calories: 318; Total Fat: 13g; Protein: 27g; Carbohydrates: 23g; Sugars: 3g; Fiber: 4g; Sodium: 496mg

Open-Faced Tuna Melts

Carbs per serving: 28g

3 SERVINGS (2 MUFFIN HALVES, TOPPED = 1 SERVING)
PREP TIME: 5 minutes | **COOK TIME:** 5 minutes

No need to fear tuna during pregnancy—just be sure to purchase canned chunk-light tuna, which is lower in mercury than albacore tuna. You'll love this warm and satisfying tuna melt.

3 English muffins, 100% whole-wheat

2 (5-ounce) cans chunk-light tuna, drained

3 tablespoons plain low-fat Greek yogurt

½ teaspoon freshly ground black pepper

¾ cup shredded Cheddar cheese

1. If your broiler is in the top of your oven, place the oven rack in the center position. Turn the broiler on high.

2. Split the English muffins, if necessary, and toast them in the toaster.

3. Meanwhile, in a medium bowl, mix the tuna, yogurt, and pepper.

4. Place the muffin halves on a baking sheet, and spoon one-sixth of the tuna mixture and 2 tablespoons of Cheddar cheese on top of each half. Broil for 2 minutes or until the cheese melts.

INGREDIENT TIP: Safe Catch is a good brand that tests and meets the low-mercury standard for pregnant women.

COMPLETE THE MEAL: Although this recipe could be consumed as a stand-alone meal, feel free to pair it with ½ cup berries, 1 small whole fruit, or ½ cup of your favorite low-sodium tomato soup.

NUTRITIONAL INFORMATION: Calories: 392; Total Fat: 13g; Protein: 40g; Carbohydrates: 28g; Sugars: 6g; Fiber: 5g; Sodium: 474mg

Pulled Pork Sandwiches

Carbs per serving: 34g

4 SERVINGS | **PREP TIME:** 5 minutes | **COOK TIME:** 15 minutes

Pulled pork sandwiches are always a hit, but the secret ingredient here is the apricot jelly. These ingredients work very well together, providing a distinctive umami flavor along with all of the nutrients you need for a balanced meal.

Avocado oil cooking spray

8 ounces store-bought pulled pork

½ cup chopped green bell pepper

2 slices provolone cheese

4 sandwich thins, 100% whole-wheat

2½ tablespoons apricot jelly

1. Heat the pulled pork according to the package instructions.

2. Heat a medium skillet over medium-low heat. When hot, coat the cooking surface with cooking spray.

3. Put the bell pepper in the skillet and cook for 5 minutes. Transfer to a small bowl and set aside.

4. Meanwhile, tear each slice of cheese into 2 strips, and halve the sandwich thins so you have a top and bottom.

5. Reduce the heat to low, and place the sandwich thins in the skillet cut-side down to toast, about 2 minutes.

6. Remove the sandwich thins from the skillet. Spread one-quarter of the jelly on the bottom half of each sandwich thin, then place one-quarter of the cheese, pulled pork, and pepper on top. Cover with the top half of the sandwich thin.

INGREDIENT TIP: Pulled pork is always a treat. Save any remaining pork for a quick taco snack, or add it to soups or salads.

NUTRITIONAL INFORMATION: Calories: 247; Total Fat: 8g; Protein: 16g; Carbohydrates: 34g; Sugars: 8g; Fiber: 6g; Sodium: 508mg

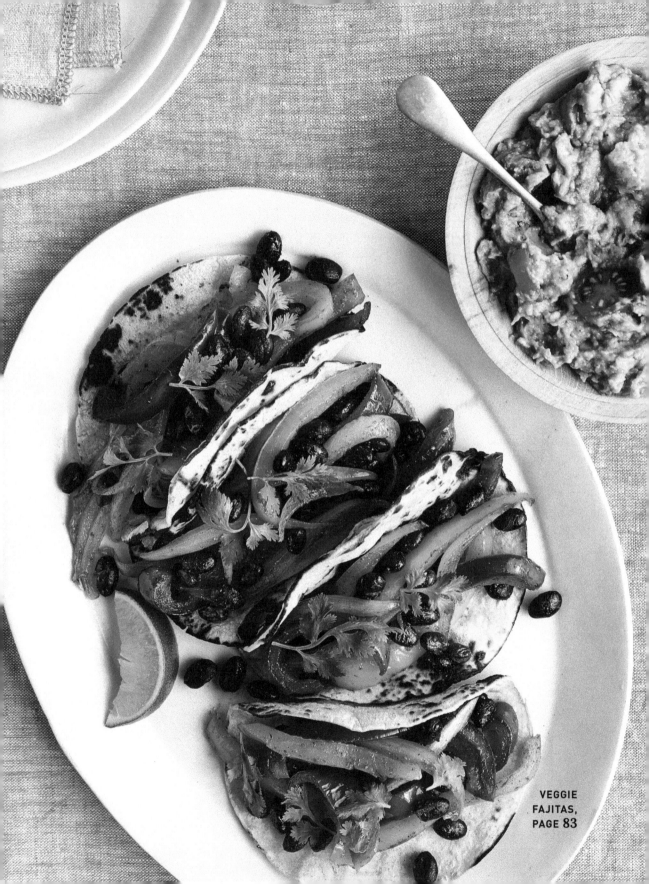

VEGGIE FAJITAS, PAGE 83

— CHAPTER FIVE —

Vegetarian

Cauliflower Steaks

Carbs per serving: 14g

---

4 SERVINGS | **PREP TIME:** 5 minutes | **COOK TIME:** 20 minutes

---

Cauliflower steaks are great because they pair well with many flavors and they're easy to prepare. You can throw them in the oven while you focus on the rest of the meal. Because cauliflower has a mild taste, I like to serve it with a sauce or dressing. This dressing is tangy and sweet and complements the arugula topping well, but you can choose whatever sauce you prefer.

FOR THE CAULIFLOWER

1 head cauliflower

Avocado oil cooking spray

½ teaspoon garlic powder

4 cups arugula

FOR THE DRESSING

1½ tablespoons honey mustard

1½ tablespoons extra-virgin olive oil

1 teaspoon freshly squeezed lemon juice

TO MAKE THE CAULIFLOWER

1. Preheat the oven to 425°F.

2. Remove the leaves from the cauliflower head, and cut it in half lengthwise.

3. Cut 1½-inch-thick steaks from each half.

4. Spray both sides of each steak with cooking spray, and season both sides with garlic powder.

5. Place the cauliflower steaks on a baking sheet, cover with foil, and roast for 10 minutes.

6. Remove the baking sheet from the oven and gently pull back the foil to avoid the steam. Flip the steaks, then roast uncovered for 10 minutes more.

7. Divide the cauliflower steaks into four equal portions. Top each portion with one-quarter of the arugula and dressing.

TO MAKE THE DRESSING

In a small bowl, whisk together the honey mustard, olive oil, and lemon juice.

COMPLETE THE MEAL: Cauliflower Steaks pair well with any protein-based dish, such as Fish Tacos (page 128) or Creamy Garlic Chicken with Broccoli (page 105).

NUTRITIONAL INFORMATION: Calories: 115; Total Fat: 6g; Protein: 5g; Carbohydrates: 14g; Sugars: 6g; Fiber: 4g; Sodium: 97mg

Veggie Fajitas

Carbs per serving: 30g

4 SERVINGS (1 FAJITA = 1 SERVING) | **PREP TIME:** 10 minutes | **COOK TIME:** 15 minutes

Have you ever tried fajitas without meat? They're just as good because the flavors in fajitas come mainly from the bell peppers and the seasoning. A friend made these for me, and I was surprised they didn't taste any different and were just as filling. These are a regular at her house, and they have become a favorite at mine, too.

FOR THE GUACAMOLE

2 small avocados pitted and peeled

1 teaspoon freshly squeezed lime juice

¼ teaspoon salt

9 cherry tomatoes, halved

FOR THE FAJITAS

1 red bell pepper

1 green bell pepper

1 small white onion

Avocado oil cooking spray

1 cup canned low-sodium black beans, drained and rinsed

½ teaspoon ground cumin

¼ teaspoon chili powder

¼ teaspoon garlic powder

4 (6-inch) yellow corn tortillas

TO MAKE THE GUACAMOLE

1. In a medium bowl, use a fork to mash the avocados with the lime juice and salt.

2. Gently stir in the cherry tomatoes.

TO MAKE THE FAJITAS

1. Cut the red bell pepper, green bell pepper, and onion into ½-inch slices.

2. Heat a large skillet over medium heat. When hot, coat the cooking surface with cooking spray. Put the peppers, onion, and beans into the skillet.

3. Add the cumin, chili powder, and garlic powder, and stir.

4. Cover and cook for 15 minutes, stirring halfway through.

5. Divide the fajita mixture equally between the tortillas, and top with guacamole and any preferred garnishes.

OPTION: Garnish with shredded Cheddar cheese, or add 4 ounces of chicken, pork, beef, or legumes for added protein.

NUTRITIONAL INFORMATION: Calories: 269; Total Fat: 15g; Protein: 8g; Carbohydrates: 30g; Sugars: 5g; Fiber: 11g; Sodium: 175mg

Easy Everyday Veggie Bowl

Carbs per serving: 35g

---

4 SERVINGS | **PREP TIME:** 5 minutes | **COOK TIME:** 30 minutes

---

This veggie bowl uses common vegetables that are available year-round and that you most likely keep on hand. This go-to meal has a very short prep time and a largely unattended cook time, so it's perfect for nights when you need a quick, filling, and nutritious dinner. Leftovers also make a tasty lunch.

---

2 small gold potatoes, cut into 1-inch dice

4 cups fresh broccoli florets

4 cups fresh cauliflower florets

4 carrots, peeled and cut into 1-inch rounds

2 tablespoons extra-virgin olive oil

4 hardboiled eggs

⅔ cup Creamy Dill Dressing (page 140)

1. Move the oven rack to the top position, and preheat the oven to 450°F.

2. In a large bowl, toss the potatoes, broccoli, cauliflower, and carrots with the olive oil. Put the vegetables in 1 or 2 roasting pans, and roast for about 30 minutes or until tender.

3. Peel and chop the hardboiled eggs.

4. Divide the vegetables between four bowls, and top each bowl with one-quarter of the chopped eggs and dill dressing.

COMPLETE THE MEAL: Although this meal can be eaten on its own, it pairs well with a fish recipe, such as Lemon Pepper Salmon (page 132), or with Coconut Lime Chicken (without the asparagus) (page 108).

NUTRITIONAL INFORMATION: Calories: 301; Total Fat: 13g; Protein: 15g; Carbohydrates: 35g; Sugars: 9g; Fiber: 7g; Sodium: 380mg

Roasted Vegetables with Creamy Dill Dressing

Carbs per serving: 38g

2 SERVINGS | **PREP TIME:** 10 minutes | **COOK TIME:** 35 minutes

This colorful veggie bowl is sure to impress and fill you up. Even though the carbs are on the higher end, there's enough fiber in this dish to balance them out.

1 medium sweet potato

12 to 15 Brussels sprouts, halved

6 teaspoons extra-virgin olive oil, divided

2 cups fresh cauliflower florets

1 medium zucchini

1 red bell pepper

⅓ cup Creamy Dill Dressing (page 140)

1. Preheat the oven to 425°F.

2. Peel and chop the sweet potato into 2-inch cubes.

3. In a large bowl, toss the sweet potato and Brussels sprouts in 2 teaspoons of oil, then place them in a large roasting pan and roast for 10 minutes.

4. Meanwhile, in a large bowl, toss the cauliflower in 2 teaspoons of oil. Remove the roasting pan from the oven, add the cauliflower, and roast for another 10 minutes.

5. Cut the zucchini into 1-inch rounds and the red bell pepper into 1-inch slices. In a large bowl, toss the zucchini and pepper in the remaining 2 teaspoons of oil. Remove the roasting pan from the oven, and add the zucchini and bell pepper. Roast for an additional 15 minutes.

6. Divide the vegetables into two portions, and top with the dill dressing.

LEFTOVER TIP: Save any leftover dill dressing for Greek Chickpea Salad (page 66).

COMPLETE THE MEAL: Pair this dish with 4 ounces of grilled chicken, steak, or fish.

NUTRITIONAL INFORMATION: Calories: 334; Total Fat: 17g; Protein: 12g; Carbohydrates: 38g; Sugars: 14g; Fiber: 11g; Sodium: 330mg

Ratatouille

Carbs per serving: 15g

4 SERVINGS | **PREP TIME:** 10 minutes | **COOK TIME:** 30 minutes

Ratatouille is a classic dish that is subject to many interpretations, but one thing's for sure: It's a simple way to add more vegetables to your diet. Vegetables are important during pregnancy because they're a superior source of vitamins and minerals, which play a major role in your baby's development.

4 tablespoons extra-virgin olive oil, divided

2 cups diced eggplant

1 cup diced zucchini

1 cup diced onion

1 cup chopped green bell pepper

1 (15-ounce) can no-salt-added diced tomatoes

1 teaspoon ground thyme

½ teaspoon garlic powder

Salt

Freshly ground black pepper

1. Heat a large saucepan over medium heat. When hot, heat 2 tablespoons of oil, then add the eggplant and the zucchini. Cook for 10 minutes, stirring occasionally. Watch to prevent burning because the eggplant will absorb the oil. Add the remaining 2 tablespoons of oil as necessary.

2. Add the onion and bell pepper, and cook for 5 minutes.

3. Add the diced tomatoes with their juices, thyme, and garlic powder, and cook for 15 minutes. Season with salt and pepper.

OPTION: Top with grated Parmesan cheese or add 1 cup chickpeas (or other preferred bean) for added protein.

INGREDIENT TIP: Save time by using frozen chopped green bell peppers instead. Cook them first over high heat with no oil until the water evaporates, then reduce the heat and proceed with the instructions.

COMPLETE THE MEAL: If you do not add beans, you can pair it with a meat, fish, or poultry dish, such as Greek Chicken Stuffed Peppers (page 106) or Roasted Pork Loin (page 114), to get adequate protein.

NUTRITIONAL INFORMATION: Calories: 190; Total Fat: 14g; Protein: 3g; Carbohydrates: 15g; Sugars: 8g; Fiber: 4g; Sodium: 28mg

Mushroom and Cauliflower Rice Risotto

Carbs per serving: 8g

---

4 SERVINGS | **PREP TIME:** 5 minutes | **COOK TIME:** 10 minutes

---

You might be surprised to learn that you don't need rice to enjoy risotto. This recipe proves it. Traditional risotto is high in carbohydrates. Replacing the rice with cauliflower not only lowers the carbs but also saves you the long cooking time.

---

1 teaspoon extra-virgin olive oil

½ cup chopped portobello mushrooms

4 cups cauliflower rice

¼ cup low-sodium vegetable broth

½ cup half-and-half

1 cup shredded Parmesan cheese

1. Heat the oil in a medium skillet over medium-low heat. When hot, put the mushrooms in the skillet and cook for 3 minutes, stirring once.

2. Add the cauliflower rice, broth, and half-and-half. Stir and cover. Increase to high heat and boil for 5 minutes.

3. Add the cheese. Stir to incorporate. Cook for 3 more minutes.

COMPLETE THE MEAL: This dish pairs beautifully with Creamy Cod with Asparagus (page 130) or Lemon Pepper Salmon (page 132), both of which will provide added protein.

NUTRITIONAL INFORMATION: Calories: 168; Total Fat: 11g; Protein: 12g; Carbohydrates: 8g; Sugars: 4g; Fiber: 3g; Sodium: 327mg

GLUTEN-FREE, VEGETARIAN, NUT-FREE

Cauli-Flowing Sweet Potato

Carbs per serving: 30g

---

4 SERVINGS (½ SWEET POTATO, TOPPED = 1 SERVING) | **PREP TIME:** 5 minutes
| **COOK TIME:** 30 minutes

If you miss loaded baked potatoes, this is the recipe for you. Sweet potatoes have less of an impact on blood sugar than russet potatoes, but portioning them is still necessary, particularly when you might be eating them with another high-carb item, like the beans in this recipe. But because beans are high in protein, they're a beneficial addition to this dish.

---

4 cups fresh cauliflower florets, cut into 2-inch pieces

2 tablespoons olive oil

2 small sweet potatoes

1 cup canned low-sodium black beans, drained and rinsed

4 lime wedges

1 cup Creamy Avocado Dressing (page 139)

1. Move the oven rack to the top position, and preheat the oven to 425°F.

2. In a large bowl, toss the cauliflower with the oil.

3. Puncture each sweet potato with a fork four times.

4. Place the cauliflower and sweet potatoes on a baking sheet. Bake for 30 minutes or until tender.

5. In the last 5 minutes of baking, microwave the beans for up to 2 minutes to warm.

6. Cut the sweet potatoes lengthwise. Top with the beans and cauliflower. Squeeze a lime wedge over each serving, and top with the avocado dressing.

COMPLETE THE MEAL: Add 4 ounces of grilled chicken for more protein.

NUTRITIONAL INFORMATION: Calories: 254; Total Fat: 10g; Protein: 11g; Carbohydrates: 30g; Sugars: 7g; Fiber: 12g; Sodium: 173mg

Stuffed Portobello Mushrooms

Carbs per serving: 12g

4 SERVINGS (2 MUSHROOMS, STUFFED = 1 SERVING) | **PREP TIME:** 5 minutes
| **COOK TIME:** 20 minutes

Portobellos are large, meaty mushrooms that go equally well in delicate Asian-inspired cuisine or with a savory beef dish. In this recipe, portobellos take the starring role. With only four simple supporting ingredients, you'd never expect the deep flavor this dish delivers. You can add a green or yellow bell pepper for more bulk and flavor, if you wish.

8 large portobello mushrooms

3 teaspoons extra-virgin olive oil, divided

4 cups fresh spinach

1 medium red bell pepper, diced

¼ cup crumbled feta

1. Preheat the oven to 450°F.

2. Remove the stems from the mushrooms, and gently scoop out the gills and discard. Coat the mushrooms with 2 teaspoons of olive oil.

3. On a baking sheet, place the mushrooms cap-side down, and roast for 20 minutes.

4. Meanwhile, heat the remaining 1 teaspoon of olive oil in a medium skillet over medium heat. When hot, sauté the spinach and red bell pepper for 8 to 10 minutes, stirring occasionally.

5. Remove the mushrooms from the oven. Drain, if necessary. Spoon the spinach and pepper mix into the mushrooms, and top with feta.

COMPLETE THE MEAL: These mushrooms are a great side dish to many recipes, including Peppered Chicken with Balsamic Kale (page 102) and Roasted Pork Loin (page 114).

NUTRITIONAL INFORMATION: Calories: 116; Total Fat: 6g; Protein: 7g; Carbohydrates: 12g; Sugars: 6g; Fiber: 4g; Sodium: 126mg

Easy Pad Thai

Carbs per serving: 25g

4 SERVINGS | **PREP TIME:** 5 minutes | **COOK TIME:** 20 minutes

Noodles are a staple in many cultures, but since they are often made from flour, they can be hard to work into your GDM management plan. Not to worry—these days, there are many low-carb noodle substitutes that allow you to keep enjoying your favorite dishes. Spiralized carrot noodles are great in this take on pad Thai—not only are they heartier than some other substitutes, but the flavors are a perfect match.

Avocado oil cooking spray

4 cups carrot noodles

4 cups fresh broccoli florets

3 ounces extra-firm tofu, cut to ½-inch cubes

⅔ cup Thai-Style Peanut Sauce (page 145)

½ cup chopped unsalted peanuts

¼ cup chopped scallions, for garnish (optional)

1. Heat a large skillet over medium-low heat. When hot, coat the cooking surface with cooking spray. Put the carrot noodles and broccoli in the skillet, and cook for 10 minutes, covered.

2. Meanwhile, press the tofu between layers of paper towels to remove any excess moisture. Be sure not to break or crumble the tofu.

3. Heat another skillet over medium heat. When hot, coat the cooking surface with cooking spray. Put the tofu in the skillet, and cook for 2 minutes on each side, until golden brown.

4. When the vegetables are tender, add the peanut sauce and toss. Divide the vegetable mixture into four equal portions, and top each portion with one-quarter of the tofu.

5. Top with the chopped peanuts and scallions (if using).

OPTION: Top with ½ cup edamame.

NUTRITIONAL INFORMATION: Calories: 419; Total Fat: 31g; Protein: 18g; Carbohydrates: 25g; Sugars: 11g; Fiber: 10g; Sodium: 323mg

Edamame Peanut Bowl

Carbs per serving: 25g

4 SERVINGS | **PREP TIME:** 5 minutes | **COOK TIME:** 15 minutes

You can eat this versatile dish hot or cold, cooked or uncooked. (Did you know raw vegetables are more filling than cooked vegetables?) If you try it raw, microwave the sauce a bit to allow it to better coat the vegetables. Top this dish with sprouts or scallions for added crunch.

2 cups frozen broccoli florets

2 cups frozen cauliflower florets

1 cup frozen shelled edamame

2 cups carrot noodles

½ cup Thai-Style Peanut Sauce (page 145)

1. Heat a large skillet over medium-high heat. When hot, add the broccoli, cauliflower, edamame, and carrot noodles, and cover. Cook for 3 to 5 minutes.

2. Uncover and cook until any water evaporates completely. The bottom of the pan should be dry when you stir.

3. Divide the vegetables into four equal portions, and top each serving with 2 tablespoons of peanut sauce.

OPTION: Microwave the frozen vegetables according to the package instructions to save time.

NUTRITIONAL INFORMATION: Calories: 283; Total Fat: 15g; Protein: 12g; Carbohydrates: 25g; Sugars: 10g; Fiber: 10g; Sodium: 172mg

No-Tuna Lettuce Wraps

Carbs per serving: 20g

4 SERVINGS | **PREP TIME:** 10 minutes

If you're uncertain about eating tuna while pregnant but you miss it, this is the recipe for you. You can even add nori to really bump up the seafood flavor. Plus, lettuce wraps are a great make-ahead for a meal or snack. If you prefer romaine or green leaf lettuce, they also work well in this recipe.

1 (15-ounce) can low-sodium chickpeas, drained and rinsed

1 celery stalk, thinly sliced

3 tablespoons honey mustard

2 tablespoons finely chopped red onion

2 tablespoons unsalted tahini

1 tablespoon capers, undrained

12 butter lettuce leaves

1. In a large bowl, mash the chickpeas.

2. Add the celery, honey mustard, onion, tahini, and capers, and mix well.

3. For each serving, place three lettuce leaves on a plate so they overlap, top with one-fourth of the chickpea filling, and roll up into a wrap. Repeat with the remaining lettuce leaves and filling.

COMPLETE THE MEAL: Have this dish with 1 to 2 hardboiled eggs or ¼ cup baby carrots with 2 tablespoons hummus for a balanced meal.

NUTRITIONAL INFORMATION: Calories: 183; Total Fat: 7g; Protein: 10g; Carbohydrates: 20g; Sugars: 9g; Fiber: 3g; Sodium: 172mg

Italian Zucchini Boats

Carbs per serving: 20g

4 SERVINGS (½ ZUCCHINI, FILLED = 1 SERVING) | **PREP TIME:** 5 minutes | **COOK TIME:** 15 minutes

I love this dish because it requires hardly any time or effort. You can jazz it up a bit by adding more vegetables, or meat, to make it a stand-alone meal. Some vegetables that complement zucchini are red bell pepper, mushrooms, and cauliflower. Each of these is low-carb, and since one zucchini boat is 20 grams of carbs, you don't have to worry about exceeding your limit.

1 cup canned low-sodium chickpeas, drained and rinsed

1 cup no-sugar-added spaghetti sauce

2 zucchini

¼ cup shredded Parmesan cheese

1. Preheat the oven to 425°F.

2. In a medium bowl, mix the chickpeas and spaghetti sauce together.

3. Cut the zucchini in half lengthwise, and scrape a spoon gently down the length of each half to remove the seeds.

4. Fill each zucchini half with the chickpea sauce, and top with one-quarter of the Parmesan cheese.

5. Place the zucchini halves on a baking sheet and roast in the oven for 15 minutes.

COMPLETE THE MEAL: This is a great side dish for meals such as Tuna Casserole (page 135) and Baked Turkey Spaghetti (page 111).

NUTRITIONAL INFORMATION: Calories: 139; Total Fat: 4g; Protein: 8g; Carbohydrates: 20g; Sugars: 6g; Fiber: 5g; Sodium: 344mg

Chickpea and Tofu Bolognese

Carbs per serving: 42g

4 SERVINGS | **PREP TIME:** 5 minutes | **COOK TIME:** 25 minutes

Tofu is a great low-carb protein to replace meat, especially in a dish like this because the texture is similar to ground beef or turkey. It takes on the flavor of whatever it is cooked with, making tofu an incredibly versatile ingredient. The second protein in this dish is chickpeas, which are also mild in flavor, so make sure the spaghetti sauce you use includes robust flavors, like garlic, basil, or oregano.

1 (3- to 4-pound) spaghetti squash

½ teaspoon ground cumin

1 cup no-sugar-added spaghetti sauce

1 (15-ounce) can low-sodium chickpeas, drained and rinsed

6 ounces extra-firm tofu

1. Preheat the oven to 400°F.

2. Cut the squash in half lengthwise. Scoop out the seeds and discard.

3. Season both halves of the squash with the cumin, and place them on a baking sheet cut-side down. Roast for 25 minutes.

4. Meanwhile, heat a medium saucepan over low heat, and pour in the spaghetti sauce and chickpeas.

5. Press the tofu between two layers of paper towels, and gently squeeze out any excess water.

6. Crumble the tofu into the sauce and cook for 15 minutes.

7. Remove the squash from the oven, and comb through the flesh of each half with a fork to make thin strands.

8. Divide the "spaghetti" into four portions, and top each portion with one-quarter of the sauce.

SUBSTITUTION TIP: Replace the spaghetti squash with any spiralized vegetable noodle and cook per the package instructions.

NUTRITIONAL INFORMATION: Calories: 275; Total Fat: 7g; Protein: 14g; Carbohydrates: 42g; Sugars: 7g; Fiber: 10g; Sodium: 55mg

Chickpea Coconut Curry

Carbs per serving: 30g

---

4 SERVINGS | **PREP TIME:** 5 minutes | **COOK TIME:** 15 minutes

---

This curry is so rich and comforting that it feels like being wrapped in a warm blanket. And what comfort food comes with such great nutrition? This dish is loaded with vitamin C from the cauliflower, calcium from the almond milk, and healthy fats from both milks.

---

3 cups fresh or frozen cauliflower florets

2 cups unsweetened almond milk

1 (15-ounce) can coconut milk

1 (15-ounce) can low-sodium chickpeas, drained and rinsed

1 tablespoon curry powder

¼ teaspoon ground ginger

¼ teaspoon garlic powder

⅛ teaspoon onion powder

¼ teaspoon salt

1. In a large stockpot, combine the cauliflower, almond milk, coconut milk, chickpeas, curry, ginger, garlic powder, and onion powder. Stir and cover.

2. Cook over medium-high heat for 10 minutes.

3. Reduce the heat to low, stir, and cook for 5 minutes more, uncovered. Season with up to ¼ teaspoon salt.

COMPLETE THE MEAL: Pair with a side salad, such as Chicken Salad Salad (page 100), for added protein and a proper amount of carbs.

NUTRITIONAL INFORMATION: Calories: 410; Total Fat: 30g; Protein: 10g; Carbohydrates: 30g; Sugars: 6g; Fiber: 9g; Sodium: 118mg

Tofu and Bean Chili

Carbs per serving: 29g

4 SERVINGS | **PREP TIME:** 10 minutes | **COOK TIME:** 30 minutes

Sometimes food aversions during pregnancy really get the best of us. Meat is a common one, either during the first trimester or throughout the entire pregnancy. In this dish, tofu works well as a ground meat replacement, which is helpful if meat is one your food aversions.

1 (15-ounce) can low-sodium dark red kidney beans, drained and rinsed, divided

2 (15-ounce) cans no-salt-added diced tomatoes

1½ cups low-sodium vegetable broth

½ teaspoon chili powder

½ teaspoon ground cumin

½ teaspoon garlic powder

½ teaspoon dried oregano

¼ teaspoon onion powder

¼ teaspoon salt

8 ounces extra-firm tofu

1. In a small bowl, mash ⅓ of the beans with a fork.

2. Put the mashed beans, the remaining whole beans, and the diced tomatoes with their juices in a large stockpot.

3. Add the broth, chili powder, cumin, garlic powder, dried oregano, onion powder, and salt. Simmer over medium-high heat for 15 minutes.

4. Press the tofu between 3 or 4 layers of paper towels to squeeze out any excess moisture.

5. Crumble the tofu into the stockpot and stir. Simmer for another 10 to 15 minutes.

OPTION: Top with any combination of garnishes, including finely diced jalapeño pepper, shredded Cheddar cheese, sliced avocado, or diced red onion.

MAKE-AHEAD TIP: Make this chili over the weekend or the night before. The flavor improves as the chili rests.

NUTRITIONAL INFORMATION: Calories: 203; Total Fat: 3g; Protein: 15g; Carbohydrates: 29g; Sugars: 10g; Fiber: 5g; Sodium: 249mg

Farro Bowl

Carbs per serving: 32g

---

4 SERVINGS | **PREP TIME:** 5 minutes | **COOK TIME:** 25 minutes

---

Farro is a type of wheat that is high in fiber, so it won't spike your blood sugar like other grains. Its nutty flavor will add a satisfying depth to your meal. Farro is a good substitute for white and brown rice. It's also a good source of vitamin B_3, which helps you metabolize proteins, carbs, and fats.

---

3 cups water

1 cup uncooked farro

1 tablespoon extra-virgin olive oil

1 teaspoon ground cumin

½ teaspoon salt

½ teaspoon freshly ground black pepper

4 hardboiled eggs, sliced

1 avocado, sliced

⅓ cup plain low-fat Greek yogurt

4 lemon wedges

1. In a medium saucepan, bring the water to a boil over high heat.

2. Pour the farro into the boiling water, and stir to submerge the grains. Reduce the heat to medium and cook for 20 minutes. Drain and set aside.

3. Heat a medium skillet over medium-low heat. When hot, pour in the oil, then add the cooked farro, cumin, salt, and pepper. Cook for 3 to 5 minutes, stirring occasionally.

4. Divide the farro into four equal portions, and top each with one-quarter of the eggs, avocado, and yogurt. Add a squeeze of lemon over the top of each portion.

COMPLETE THE MEAL: Although this meal can be consumed on its own, feel free to include additional protein, such as 4 ounces of grilled or baked chicken or fish.

NUTRITIONAL INFORMATION: Calories: 332; Total Fat: 16g; Protein: 15g; Carbohydrates: 32g; Sugars: 2g; Fiber: 8g; Sodium: 359mg

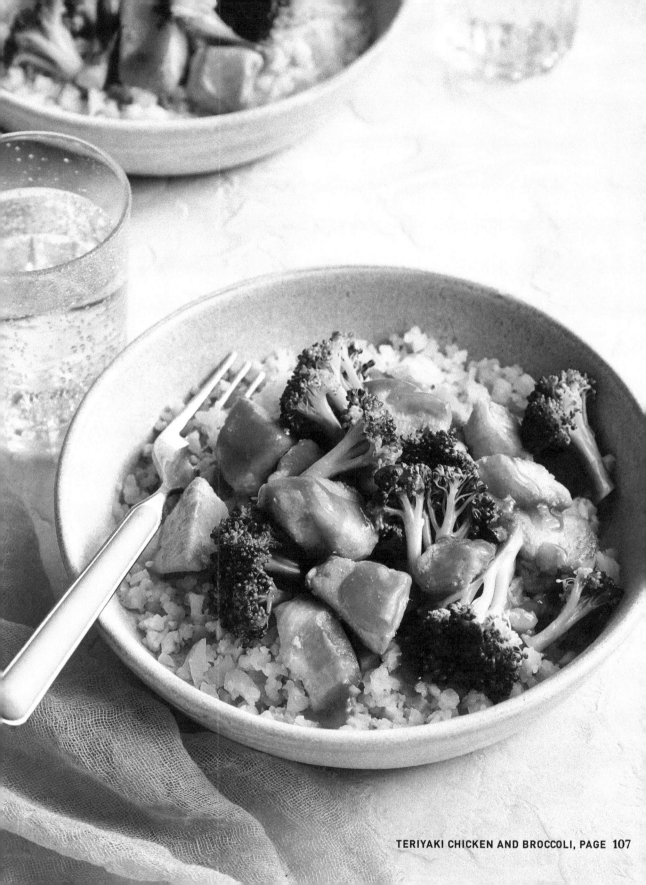

TERIYAKI CHICKEN AND BROCCOLI, PAGE 107

Poultry

Chicken Salad Salad

Carbs per serving: 10g

4 SERVINGS | PREP TIME: 15 minutes

For this no-cook lunch, simply layer chicken salad over a bed of lettuce. Ingredients like celery, scallions, parsley, and cucumber can be added in any combination to vary the flavors and texture of this salad. Or, if you aren't opposed to nuts, try adding ¼ cup chopped pecans in the second step to add crunch.

2 cups shredded rotisserie chicken

1½ tablespoons plain low-fat Greek yogurt

⅛ teaspoon freshly ground black pepper

¼ cup halved purple seedless grapes

8 cups chopped romaine lettuce

1 medium tomato, sliced

1 avocado, sliced

1. In a large bowl, combine the chicken, yogurt, and pepper, and mix well.

2. Stir in the grapes.

3. Divide the lettuce into four portions. Spoon one-quarter of the chicken salad onto each portion and top with a couple slices of tomato and avocado.

COMPLETE THE MEAL: Pair this protein-rich salad with a vegetarian side dish, such as Chickpea Coconut Curry (page 95) or Italian Zucchini Boats (page 93), to increase your carbs and fiber.

NUTRITIONAL INFORMATION: Calories: 203; Total Fat: 10g; Protein: 22g; Carbohydrates: 10g; Sugars: 4g; Fiber: 5g; Sodium: 56mg

Honey Mustard Chicken Lettuce Wraps

Carbs per serving: 8g

4 SERVINGS (2 WRAPS = 1 SERVING) | **PREP TIME:** 10 minutes

Lettuce wraps are a great way to enjoy favorites like burgers and sandwiches without the excess carbs. In most cases, by removing the bun (or bread), you've cut out the bulk of the carbohydrates, leaving only those inherent to the natural foods. This low-carb meal is packed with nutritious ingredients and can be accompanied by a small piece of whole fruit or a salad.

8 romaine lettuce leaves

1½ cups shredded rotisserie chicken

1 avocado, sliced

2 hardboiled eggs, sliced

1 medium tomato, sliced

4 teaspoons honey mustard

1. Top each lettuce leaf with one-eighth of the chicken, avocado, eggs, and tomato.

2. Drizzle the honey mustard over the filling, and working from the edge closest to you, roll up each lettuce leaf to make the wraps.

LEFTOVER TIP: Use leftover rotisserie chicken for Chicken Salad Salad (page 100) or Open-Faced Chicken and Onion Grilled Cheese (page 77).

NUTRITIONAL INFORMATION: Calories: 227; Total Fat: 11g; Protein: 24g; Carbohydrates: 8g; Sugars: 3g; Fiber: 4g; Sodium: 159mg

Peppered Chicken with Balsamic Kale

Carbs per serving: 18g

4 SERVINGS | **PREP TIME:** 5 minutes | **COOK TIME:** 15 minutes

Balsamic vinegar is a great ingredient because it has an umami effect, meaning it satisfies your taste buds beyond the sensations of sweet, sour, salty, and bitter. In this recipe, the vinegar adds pep to the chicken and softens the flavor and texture of the kale, which is full of important nutrients, like vitamins K and C.

4 (4-ounce) boneless, skinless chicken breasts

¼ teaspoon salt

1 tablespoon freshly ground black pepper

2 tablespoons unsalted butter

1 tablespoon extra-virgin olive oil

8 cups stemmed and roughly chopped kale, loosely packed (about 2 bunches)

½ cup balsamic vinegar

20 cherry tomatoes, halved

1. Season both sides of the chicken breasts with the salt and pepper.

2. Heat a large skillet over medium heat. When hot, heat the butter and oil. Add the chicken and cook for 8 to 10 minutes, flipping halfway through. When cooked all the way through, remove the chicken from the skillet and set aside.

3. Increase the heat to medium-high. Put the kale in the skillet and cook for 3 minutes, stirring every minute.

4. Add the vinegar and the tomatoes and cook for another 3 to 5 minutes.

5. Divide the kale and tomato mixture into four equal portions, and top each portion with 1 chicken breast.

COMPLETE THE MEAL: Pair this recipe with the Stuffed Portobello Mushrooms (page 89) or Mushroom and Cauliflower Rice Risotto (page 87) for additional carbohydrates.

NUTRITIONAL INFORMATION: Calories: 293; Total Fat: 11g; Protein: 31g; Carbohydrates: 18g; Sugars: 4g; Fiber: 3g; Sodium: 328mg

One-Pan Chicken Dinner

Carbs per serving: 23g

---

4 SERVINGS | **PREP TIME:** 5 minutes | **COOK TIME:** 35 minutes

---

Brussels sprouts are named after the capital of Belgium. They are related to cabbage and are just as versatile. They are also low in calories and packed with vitamins A and C, folic acid, fiber, and an impressive amount of protein. These little vegetables really pack a punch. Try them shaved in salads, steamed, or, as with this dish, roasted.

---

3 tablespoons extra-virgin olive oil

1 tablespoon red wine vinegar or apple cider vinegar

¼ teaspoon garlic powder

3 tablespoons Italian seasoning

4 (4-ounce) boneless, skinless chicken breasts

2 cups cubed sweet potatoes

20 Brussels sprouts, halved lengthwise

1. Preheat the oven to 400°F.

2. In a large bowl, whisk together the oil, vinegar, garlic powder, and Italian seasoning.

3. Add the chicken, sweet potatoes, and Brussels sprouts, and coat thoroughly with the marinade.

4. Remove the ingredients from the marinade and arrange them on a baking sheet in a single layer. Roast for 15 minutes.

5. Remove the baking sheet from the oven, flip the chicken over, and bake for another 15 to 20 minutes.

COMPLETE THE MEAL: This is a complete meal, but feel free to add additional nonstarchy vegetables, if desired.

NUTRITIONAL INFORMATION: Calories: 342; Total Fat: 16g; Protein: 30g; Carbohydrates: 23g; Sugars: 8g; Fiber: 9g; Sodium: 186mg

Rosemary Chicken with Potatoes and Green Beans

Carbs per serving: 38g

4 SERVINGS | **PREP TIME:** 5 minutes | **COOK TIME:** 30 minutes

This recipe will impress the family without you having to stand over the stove—just throw everything in the oven and you're on your way to a delicious meal. Potatoes are a hearty staple, but if you know your glucose doesn't respond well to them, try similar foods with lesser glucose impact, like sweet potatoes, butternut squash, farro, or quinoa. All would work well with this dish.

⅓ cup low-sodium chicken broth

¼ cup extra-virgin olive oil

½ teaspoon salt

½ teaspoon freshly ground black pepper

¼ teaspoon garlic powder

¼ teaspoon dried thyme

1 teaspoon dried rosemary

4 (4-ounce) boneless, skinless chicken breasts

4 small gold potatoes, cubed

1 pound green beans

1. Preheat the oven to 400°F.

2. In a large bowl, whisk together the broth, oil, salt, pepper, garlic powder, thyme, and rosemary.

3. Add the chicken and potatoes to the marinade and coat well. Reserving the marinade, use a slotted spoon to remove the chicken and potatoes.

4. Arrange the chicken and potatoes on a baking sheet in a single layer and roast for 15 minutes.

5. Meanwhile, trim the green bean ends, if necessary, and put the beans in the reserved marinade.

6. Remove the baking sheet from the oven, flip the chicken breasts over, and add the green beans to the baking sheet. Pour the remaining marinade over the chicken.

7. Bake for 10 to 12 minutes until the chicken is cooked through, then broil for 2 minutes for a crisp, brown crust.

INGREDIENT TIP: Green beans come in a variety of shapes and sizes—from thin, sweet haricots verts (which often come pretrimmed and packaged in the produce section) to hearty Blue Lake beans to yellow bush beans. Any would work with this dish.

NUTRITIONAL INFORMATION: Calories: 398; Total Fat: 15g; Protein: 32g; Carbohydrates: 38g; Sugars: 5g; Fiber: 8g; Sodium: 393mg

Creamy Garlic Chicken with Broccoli

Carbs per serving: 22g

4 SERVINGS | **PREP TIME:** 5 minutes | **COOK TIME:** 15 minutes

Brown rice and quinoa are both good substitutes for white rice. Even though the amount of carbohydrates is equal to white rice, they have nutritionally superior carbohydrates. Brown rice and quinoa provide fiber and protein that white rice lacks, which are better for your blood sugar.

½ cup uncooked brown rice or quinoa

4 (4-ounce) boneless, skinless chicken breasts

¼ teaspoon salt

¼ teaspoon freshly ground black pepper

1 teaspoon garlic powder, divided

Avocado oil cooking spray

3 cups fresh or frozen broccoli florets

1 cup half-and-half

1. Cook the rice according to the package instructions.

2. Meanwhile, season both sides of the chicken breasts with the salt, pepper, and ½ teaspoon of garlic powder.

3. Heat a large skillet over medium-low heat. When hot, coat the cooking surface with cooking spray and add the chicken and broccoli in a single layer.

4. Cook for 4 minutes, then flip the chicken breasts over and cover. Cook for 5 minutes more.

5. Add the half-and-half and remaining ½ teaspoon of garlic powder to the skillet and stir. Increase the heat to high and simmer for 2 minutes.

6. Divide the rice into four equal portions. Top each portion with 1 chicken breast and one-quarter of the broccoli and cream sauce.

COMPLETE THE MEAL: Although this can be a stand-alone meal, there's always room for additional vegetables.

NUTRITIONAL INFORMATION: Calories: 303; Total Fat: 10g; Protein: 33g; Carbohydrates: 22g; Sugars: 4g; Fiber: 3g; Sodium: 271mg

Greek Chicken Stuffed Peppers

Carbs per serving: 20g

---

4 SERVINGS (½ BELL PEPPER, STUFFED = 1 SERVING)
PREP TIME: 5 minutes | **COOK TIME:** 30 minutes

If you've noticed that your blood sugar doesn't respond well to grains—even higher-nutrition grains, like brown rice, quinoa, or farro—you can remove them from this meal without missing out. However, removing the grains means taking away the main source of carbs, so it may be too low-carb for your needs. If that's the case, you can incorporate carrots or a palm-size potato.

2 large red bell peppers

2 teaspoons extra-virgin olive oil, divided

½ cup uncooked brown rice or quinoa

4 (4-ounce) boneless, skinless chicken breasts

¼ teaspoon garlic powder

¼ teaspoon onion powder

⅛ teaspoon dried thyme

½ teaspoon dried oregano

½ cup crumbled feta

1. Cut the bell peppers in half and remove the seeds.

2. In a large skillet, heat 1 teaspoon of olive oil over low heat. When hot, place the bell pepper halves cut-side up in the skillet. Cover and cook for 20 minutes.

3. Cook the rice according to the package instructions.

4. Meanwhile, cut the chicken into 1-inch pieces.

5. In a medium skillet, heat the remaining 1 teaspoon of olive oil over medium-low heat. When hot, add the chicken.

6. Season the chicken with the garlic powder, onion powder, thyme, and oregano.

7. Cook for 5 minutes, stirring occasionally, until cooked through.

8. In a large bowl, combine the cooked rice and chicken. Scoop one-quarter of the chicken and rice mixture into each pepper half, cover, and cook for 10 minutes over low heat.

9. Top each pepper half with 2 tablespoons of crumbled feta.

MAKE-AHEAD TIP: If you have batch cooked your rice or quinoa in advance, you will need 1½ cups of it. For both grains, 1 cup of uncooked grain is equal to about 3 cups cooked.

COMPLETE THE MEAL: For a more filling meal, pair this dish with Ratatouille (page 86).

NUTRITIONAL INFORMATION: Calories: 288; Total Fat: 10g; Protein: 32g; Carbohydrates: 20g; Sugars: 4g; Fiber: 4g; Sodium: 267mg

Teriyaki Chicken and Broccoli

Carbs per serving: 20g

4 SERVINGS | **PREP TIME:** 5 minutes | **COOK TIME:** 20 minutes

If you're yearning for Japanese food, a simple teriyaki-style dish is a great way to satisfy your cravings. Making your own teriyaki sauce allows you to control the sodium as well as the amount and type of sugar. Low-sodium soy sauce and honey are healthier for you and your baby, and replacing white rice with cauliflower rice eliminates the possibility of a glucose spike.

FOR THE SAUCE

½ cup water

2 tablespoons low-sodium soy sauce

2 tablespoons honey

1 tablespoon rice vinegar

¼ teaspoon garlic powder

Pinch ground ginger

1 tablespoon cornstarch

FOR THE ENTRÉE

1 tablespoon sesame oil

4 (4-ounce) boneless, skinless chicken breasts, cut into bite-size cubes

1 (12-ounce) bag frozen broccoli

1 (12-ounce) bag frozen cauliflower rice

TO MAKE THE SAUCE

1. In a small saucepan, whisk together the water, soy sauce, honey, rice vinegar, garlic powder, and ginger. Add the cornstarch and whisk until it is fully incorporated.

2. Over medium heat, bring the teriyaki sauce to a boil. Let the sauce boil for 1 minute to thicken. Remove the sauce from the heat and set aside.

TO MAKE THE ENTRÉE

1. Heat a large skillet over medium-low heat. When hot, add the oil and the chicken. Cook for 5 to 7 minutes, until the chicken is cooked through, stirring as needed.

2. Steam the broccoli and cauliflower rice in the microwave according to the package instructions.

3. Divide the cauliflower rice into four equal portions. Put one-quarter of the broccoli and chicken over each portion and top with the teriyaki sauce.

COMPLETE THE MEAL: Balance this meal with shelled edamame or veggie sticks dipped in ¼ cup hummus to achieve adequate carb count.

NUTRITIONAL INFORMATION: Calories: 247; Total Fat: 7g; Protein: 29g; Carbohydrates: 20g; Sugars: 12g; Fiber: 5g; Sodium: 418mg

Coconut Lime Chicken

Carbs per serving: 11g

4 SERVINGS | **PREP TIME:** 5 minutes | **COOK TIME:** 15 minutes

Island flavors are a great break from more traditional American flavors. They bring new life to the chicken and cauliflower in this dish and taste great in the summertime. For a warm-weather dish, you can marinate the chicken and vegetables in the coconut milk and lime mixture for about an hour before cooking, then cook the chicken and vegetables on the grill.

1 tablespoon coconut oil

4 (4-ounce) boneless, skinless chicken breasts

½ teaspoon salt

1 red bell pepper, cut into ¼-inch-thick slices

16 asparagus spears, bottom ends trimmed

1 cup unsweetened coconut milk

2 tablespoons freshly squeezed lime juice

½ teaspoon garlic powder

¼ teaspoon red pepper flakes

¼ cup chopped fresh cilantro

1. In a large skillet, heat the oil over medium-low heat. When hot, add the chicken.

2. Season the chicken with the salt. Cook for 5 minutes, then flip.

3. Push the chicken to the side of the skillet, and add the bell pepper and asparagus. Cook, covered, for 5 minutes.

4. Meanwhile, in a small bowl, whisk together the coconut milk, lime juice, garlic powder, and red pepper flakes.

5. Add the coconut milk mixture to the skillet, and boil over high heat for 2 to 3 minutes.

6. Top with the cilantro.

COMPLETE THE MEAL: This recipe is very low in carbs, so pair it with a vegetable recipe, such as Cauliflower Leek Soup (page 60), Kidney Bean Salad (page 68), or the Easy Everyday Veggie Bowl (page 84).

NUTRITIONAL INFORMATION: Calories: 321; Total Fat: 19g; Protein: 30g; Carbohydrates: 11g; Sugars: 6g; Fiber: 4g; Sodium: 378mg

Taco Stuffed Sweet Potatoes

Carbs per serving: 27g

4 SERVINGS (2 POTATO HALVES, STUFFED = 1 SERVING)
PREP TIME: 5 minutes | **COOK TIME:** 15 minutes

Ground turkey and sweet potatoes are a magical pairing in this Mexican-inspired dish. Top the potatoes with any combination of your favorite garnishes, such as shredded Cheddar cheese, sliced avocado, sour cream, finely diced jalapeño pepper, chopped cilantro, or pico de gallo.

4 medium sweet potatoes

2 tablespoons extra-virgin olive oil

1 pound 93% lean ground turkey

2 teaspoons ground cumin

1 teaspoon chili powder

½ teaspoon salt

½ teaspoon freshly ground black pepper

1. Pierce the potatoes with a fork, and microwave them on the potato setting, or for 10 minutes on high power.

2. Meanwhile, heat a medium skillet over medium heat. When hot, put the oil, turkey, cumin, chili powder, salt, and pepper into the skillet, stirring and breaking apart the meat, as needed.

3. Remove the potatoes from the microwave and halve them lengthwise. Depress the centers with a spoon, and fill each half with an equal amount of cooked turkey.

COMPLETE THE MEAL: Pair with a serving of your favorite vegetable, such as broccoli, carrots, or corn.

NUTRITIONAL INFORMATION: Calories: 300g; Total Fat: 8g; Protein: 30g; Carbohydrates: 27g; Sugars: 4g; Fiber: 5g; Sodium: 426mg

Chicken Enchilada Spaghetti Squash

Carbs per serving: 17g

4 SERVINGS | PREP TIME: 5 minutes | COOK TIME: 40 minutes

We've merged two meals here—chicken enchiladas and low-carb spaghetti—for a dish with a new spin. Enchiladas and spaghetti are high-carb, but in this dish, the carbohydrates are replaced with low-carb spaghetti squash.

1 (3-pound) spaghetti squash, halved lengthwise and seeded

1½ teaspoons ground cumin, divided

Avocado oil cooking spray

4 (4-ounce) boneless, skinless chicken breasts

1 large zucchini, diced

¾ cup canned red enchilada sauce

¾ cup shredded Cheddar or mozzarella cheese

1. Preheat the oven to 400°F.

2. Season both halves of the squash with ½ teaspoon of cumin, and place them cut-side down on a baking sheet. Bake for 25 to 30 minutes.

3. Meanwhile, heat a large skillet over medium-low heat. When hot, spray the cooking surface with cooking spray and add the chicken breasts, zucchini, and 1 teaspoon of cumin. Cook the chicken for 4 to 5 minutes per side. Stir the zucchini when you flip the chicken.

4. Transfer the zucchini to a medium bowl and set aside. Remove the chicken from the skillet, and let it rest for 10 minutes or until it's cool enough to handle. Shred or dice the cooked chicken.

5. Place the chicken and zucchini in a large bowl, and add the enchilada sauce.

6. Remove the squash from the oven, flip it over, and comb through it with a fork to make thin strands.

7. Scoop the chicken mixture on top of the squash halves and top with the cheese. Return the squash to the oven and broil for 2 to 5 minutes, or until the cheese is bubbly.

COMPLETE THE MEAL: Serve with a vegetable side dish, such as Cauliflower Steaks (page 82) or a vegetarian version of Slow Cooker Ropa Vieja (page 123)—simply omit the meat.

NUTRITIONAL INFORMATION: Calories: 331; Total Fat: 11g; Protein: 35g; Carbohydrates: 27g; Sugars: 2g; Fiber: 4g; Sodium: 491mg

Baked Turkey Spaghetti

Carbs per serving: 12g

---

4 SERVINGS | **PREP TIME:** 5 minutes | **COOK TIME:** 20 minutes

---

Spaghetti is really something special when it's layered with cheese and broiled until gooey and bubbly, but it is full of empty carbs from the white-flour pasta and extra fat from the beef in meat sauces. Using ground turkey and zucchini noodles gives you a healthier meal that will still satisfy your spaghetti craving.

---

1 (10-ounce) package zucchini noodles

2 tablespoons extra-virgin olive oil, divided

1 pound 93% lean ground turkey

½ teaspoon dried oregano

2 cups low-sodium spaghetti sauce

½ cup shredded sharp Cheddar cheese

1. Pat zucchini noodles dry between two paper towels.

2. In an oven-safe medium skillet, heat 1 tablespoon of olive oil over medium heat. When hot, add the zucchini noodles. Cook for 3 minutes, stirring halfway through.

3. Add the remaining 1 tablespoon of oil, ground turkey, and oregano. Cook for 7 to 10 minutes, stirring and breaking apart, as needed.

4. Add the spaghetti sauce to the skillet and stir.

5. If your broiler is in the top of your oven, place the oven rack in the center position. Set the broiler on high.

6. Top the mixture with the cheese, and broil for 5 minutes or until the cheese is bubbly.

COMPLETE THE MEAL: Pair with Ratatouille (page 86) or Italian Zucchini Boats (page 93) to achieve the right amount of carbs.

NUTRITIONAL INFORMATION: Calories: 335; Total Fat: 21g; Protein: 28g; Carbohydrates: 12g; Sugars: 4g; Fiber: 3g; Sodium: 216mg

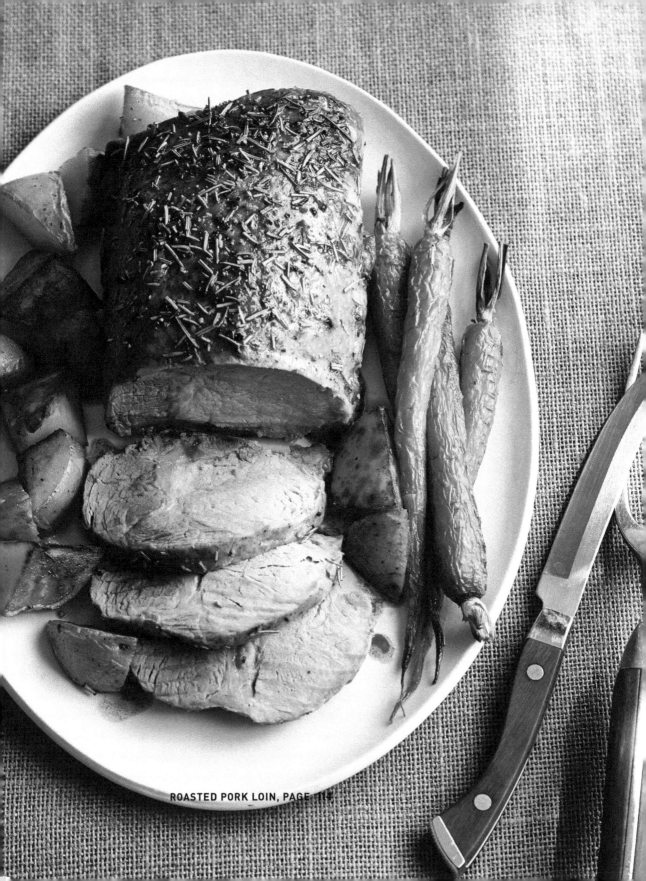

ROASTED PORK LOIN, PAGE 114

— CHAPTER SEVEN —

Beef, Pork, Lamb

Roasted Pork Loin

Carbs per serving: 26g

4 SERVINGS | **PREP TIME:** 5 minutes | **COOK TIME:** 40 minutes, plus 10 minutes to rest

Rosemary is a magical herb that will give your dinner the extra oomph you're looking for. It's fabulous with pork, potatoes, and carrots, which is why all three are included in this one-pot meal. If you'd like a bigger serving of potatoes, you can swap the gold potatoes for lower-carb sweet potatoes.

1 pound pork loin

1 tablespoon extra-virgin olive oil, divided

2 teaspoons honey

¼ teaspoon freshly ground black pepper

½ teaspoon dried rosemary

2 small gold potatoes, chopped into 2-inch cubes

4 (6-inch) carrots, chopped into ½-inch rounds

1. Preheat the oven to 350°F.

2. Rub the pork loin with ½ tablespoon of oil and the honey. Season with the pepper and rosemary.

3. In a medium bowl, toss the potatoes and carrots in the remaining ½ tablespoon of oil.

4. Place the pork and the vegetables on a baking sheet in a single layer. Cook for 40 minutes.

5. Remove the baking sheet from the oven and let the pork rest for at least 10 minutes before slicing. Divide the pork and vegetables into four equal portions.

LEFTOVER TIP: You'll likely have to purchase a 2-pound pork loin. Cook the whole loin, and use half for this recipe. Save the remaining pork for Low-Carb Ramen with Pork Loin (page 64).

COMPLETE THE MEAL: This dish goes well with Summer Salad (page 65) or Cauliflower Leek Soup (page 60).

NUTRITIONAL INFORMATION: Calories: 343; Total Fat: 10g; Protein: 26g; Carbohydrates: 26g; Sugars: 6g; Fiber: 4g; Sodium: 109mg

Mediterranean Lamb Bowl

Carbs per serving: 28g

4 SERVINGS | **PREP TIME:** 10 minutes | **COOK TIME:** 10 minutes

Lamb is a high-quality protein source, rich in vitamin B_{12}, iron, and zinc. All three of these nutrients help keep you and your baby healthy and strong during pregnancy. If you cannot get lamb or it is not to your taste, 93% lean ground beef or turkey works just as well in this recipe.

1 pound lean ground lamb

¼ teaspoon onion powder

¼ teaspoon garlic powder

¼ teaspoon ground ginger

4 cups chopped romaine lettuce

1 large tomato, diced

1 medium peeled and diced cucumber

½ cup Creamy Dill Dressing (page 140)

4 sandwich thins, 100% whole-wheat, toasted

1. Heat a medium skillet over medium-low heat. When hot, put the lamb, onion powder, garlic powder, and ginger in the skillet. Break the lamb apart with a spoon, and cook for 7 to 10 minutes, or until the lamb is cooked through.

2. Meanwhile, divide the lettuce, tomato, and cucumber equally between four bowls. Add one-quarter of the lamb to each bowl.

3. Top with the dill dressing, and add a toasted sandwich thin on the side of each portion.

COMPLETE THE MEAL: Serve alongside your favorite fruit, such as ½ cup berries or grapes or 1 small apple, pear, or orange.

NUTRITIONAL INFORMATION: Calories: 435; Total Fat: 18g; Protein: 34g; Carbohydrates: 28g; Sugars: 6g; Fiber: 7g; Sodium: 419mg

Sloppy Joes

Carbs per serving: 36g

---

4 SERVINGS | **PREP TIME:** 10 minutes | **COOK TIME:** 15 minutes

---

Who says you can't enjoy the classics? Sloppy Joes are entirely acceptable with a few tweaks. The biggest adjustment is switching the bun for a bread that brings you within your appropriate carbohydrate range. Even 100% whole-wheat buns are better than regular white buns. The other notable modification is making sure you use no-sugar-added ketchup.

---

1 pound 93% lean ground beef

½ medium yellow onion, chopped

1 medium red bell pepper, chopped

1 (15-ounce) can no-salt-added tomato sauce

2 tablespoons no-salt-added, no-sugar-added ketchup

2 tablespoons low-sodium Worcestershire sauce

4 sandwich thins, 100% whole-wheat

1 cup shredded cabbage

1. Heat a large skillet over medium heat. When hot, cook the beef, onion, and bell pepper for 7 to 10 minutes, stirring and breaking apart as needed.

2. Stir in the tomato sauce, ketchup, and Worcestershire sauce. Increase the heat to medium-high and simmer for 5 minutes.

3. Cut the sandwich thins in half so there is a top and a bottom. For each serving, place one-quarter of the filling and cabbage on the bottom half, then cover with the top half.

COMPLETE THE MEAL: This is a complete and hearty meal, but feel free to pair it with your favorite vegetables on the side.

NUTRITIONAL INFORMATION: Calories: 328; Total Fat: 9g; Protein: 31g; Carbohydrates: 36g; Sugars: 11g; Fiber: 8g; Sodium: 274mg

Open-Faced Philly Cheesesteak Sandwiches

Carbs per serving: 33g

---

4 SERVINGS (2 MUFFIN HALVES, TOPPED = 1 SERVING)
PREP TIME: 5 minutes | **COOK TIME:** 25 minutes

Most would think that Philly cheesesteaks are out of the question with GDM, but you can absolutely make it work for you. No need to worry about sodium with these portions, and if you want a leaner meat, you can use 93% lean ground turkey instead. The English muffins add a chewy bread texture you'll love.

Avocado oil cooking spray

1 cup chopped yellow onion

1 green bell pepper, chopped

12 ounces 93% lean ground beef

Pinch salt

¾ teaspoon freshly ground black pepper

4 slices provolone or Swiss cheese

4 English muffins, 100% whole-wheat

1. Heat a large skillet over medium-low heat. When hot, coat the cooking surface with cooking spray, and arrange the onion and pepper in an even layer. Cook for 8 to 10 minutes, stirring every 3 to 4 minutes.

2. Push the vegetables to one side of the skillet and add the beef, breaking it into large chunks. Cook for 7 to 9 minutes, until a crisp crust forms on the bottom of the meat.

3. Season the beef with the salt and pepper, then flip the beef over and break it down into smaller chunks.

4. Stir the vegetables and the beef together, then top with the cheese and cook for 2 minutes.

5. Meanwhile, split each muffin in half, if necessary, then toast the muffins in a toaster.

6. Place one-eighth of the filling on each muffin half.

COMPLETE THE MEAL: Pair with your favorite piece of fruit, such as ½ cup berries or grapes or 1 small apple, pear, or orange.

NUTRITIONAL INFORMATION: Calories: 398; Total Fat: 16g; Protein: 31g; Carbohydrates: 33g; Sugars: 8g; Fiber: 6g; Sodium: 371mg

Cheeseburger and Cauliflower Wraps

Carbs per serving: 7g

---

4 SERVINGS | PREP TIME: 5 minutes | **COOK TIME:** 20 minutes

---

Another way to compensate for the carbs you are used to having (the bun, in this case) is to add extra flavor and texture. Mushrooms give this dish a deep, full flavor that makes the meal more complex, and the light and crisp texture of the lettuce freshens everything up. You also have room here to add more carbs. Try diced carrots and sauté them with the mushrooms, or add diced tomatoes into the wrap.

Avocado oil cooking spray

½ cup chopped white onion

1 cup chopped portobello mushrooms

1 pound 93% lean ground beef

½ teaspoon garlic powder

Pinch salt

1 (10-ounce) bag frozen cauliflower rice

12 iceberg lettuce leaves

¾ cup shredded Cheddar cheese

1. Heat a large skillet over medium heat. When hot, coat the cooking surface with cooking spray and add the onion and mushrooms. Cook for 5 minutes, stirring occasionally.

2. Add the beef, garlic powder, and salt, stirring and breaking apart the meat as needed. Cook for 5 minutes.

3. Stir in the frozen cauliflower rice and increase the heat to medium-high. Cook for 5 minutes more, or until the water evaporates.

4. For each portion, use three lettuce leaves. Spoon one-quarter of the filling onto the lettuce leaves, and top with one-quarter of the cheese. Then, working from the side closest to you, roll up the lettuce to close the wrap. Repeat with the remaining lettuce leaves and filling.

COMPLETE THE MEAL: Serve alongside a vegetable side dish, such as Stuffed Portobello Mushrooms (page 89) or Mushroom and Cauliflower Rice Risotto (page 87). Or pair with a generous helping of your favorite vegetables, cooked however you prefer.

NUTRITIONAL INFORMATION: Calories: 288; Total Fat: 15g; Protein: 31g; Carbohydrates: 7g; Sugars: 4g; Fiber: 3g; Sodium: 264mg

Steak Fajita Bake

Carbs per serving: 28g

4 SERVINGS | **PREP TIME:** 10 minutes | **COOK TIME:** 15 minutes

Veggie Fajitas (page 83) are delicious and let the vegetables shine. They are terrific when you want a lighter meal, but these fajitas give you added protein from the steak. If you don't eat red meat, you could also try this recipe with four 4-ounce boneless, skinless chicken breasts. To prepare the sirloin steak, make sure you trim all visible fat from the edges before cooking.

1 green bell pepper

1 yellow bell pepper

1 red bell pepper

1 small white onion

10 ounces sirloin steak, trimmed of visible fat

2 tablespoons avocado oil

½ teaspoon ground cumin

¼ teaspoon chili powder

¼ teaspoon garlic powder

4 (6-inch) 100% whole-wheat tortillas

1. Preheat the oven to 400°F.

2. Cut the green bell pepper, yellow bell pepper, red bell pepper, onion, and steak into ½-inch-thick slices, and put them on a large baking sheet.

3. In a small bowl, combine the oil, cumin, chili powder, and garlic powder, then drizzle the mixture over the meat and vegetables to fully coat them.

4. Arrange the steak and vegetables in a single layer, and bake for 10 to 15 minutes, or until the steak is cooked through.

5. Divide the steak and vegetables equally between the tortillas.

OPTION: Top with cheese, cilantro, or guacamole, if desired.

COMPLETE THE MEAL: Pair with a side of vegetables, such as steamed broccoli or additional sautéed bell peppers.

NUTRITIONAL INFORMATION: Calories: 349; Total Fat: 18g; Protein: 19g; Carbohydrates: 28g; Sugars: 5g; Fiber: 5g; Sodium: 197mg

Smothered Burritos

Carbs per serving: 28g

---

4 SERVINGS (2 BURRITOS = 1 SERVING) | **PREP TIME:** 5 minutes | **COOK TIME:** 20 minutes

---

Before I began cooking healthier meals, I often made this dish with pot roast and canned enchilada sauce, but when I realized how high the fat and sodium content of that combination is, I knew I had to make a change. I created a version that is just as delicious, less heavy, and much healthier than the original. If your family is anything like mine, this dish will quickly become a favorite.

Avocado oil cooking spray

½ small yellow onion, chopped

1 red bell pepper, chopped

1 pound 93% lean ground turkey

1 teaspoon dried oregano

½ teaspoon smoked paprika

½ teaspoon garlic powder

8 medium yellow corn tortillas

1¼ cups jarred salsa or pico de gallo

¾ cup shredded Cheddar cheese

1. Heat a medium skillet over medium-low heat. When hot, coat the cooking surface with cooking spray, and place the onion, pepper, and ground turkey in the skillet.

2. Season the turkey with the oregano, smoked paprika, and garlic powder, and stir. Cook for 7 minutes.

3. Spoon ¼ cup of turkey into each tortilla. Wrap each tortilla into a burrito, then place the burritos seam-side down in a casserole dish. Pour the salsa over the burritos.

4. If your broiler is in the top of your oven, set the rack in the middle position. Set the broiler to high.

5. Top the burritos with the cheese, and broil for 4 minutes, or until the cheese is melted.

NUTRITIONAL INFORMATION: Calories: 384; Total Fat: 16g; Protein: 31g; Carbohydrates: 28g; Sugars: 5g; Fiber: 4g; Sodium: 377mg

Beef Burrito Bowl

Carbs per serving: 14g

4 SERVINGS | **PREP TIME:** 5 minutes | **COOK TIME:** 15 minutes

One of the hardest things to juggle with GDM is time. Managing your life and work, planning for your baby, and making frequent visits to the doctor can take their toll. The last thing you need is to spend hours in the kitchen. With very short prep and cook times, this easy burrito bowl is a great go-to meal when you don't have a minute to spare.

1 pound 93% lean ground beef

1 cup canned low-sodium black beans, drained and rinsed

¼ teaspoon ground cumin

¼ teaspoon chili powder

¼ teaspoon garlic powder

¼ teaspoon onion powder

¼ teaspoon salt

1 head romaine or preferred lettuce, shredded

2 medium tomatoes, chopped

1 cup shredded Cheddar cheese or packaged cheese blend

1. Heat a large skillet over medium-low heat. Put the beef, beans, cumin, chili powder, garlic powder, onion powder, and salt into the skillet, and cook for 8 to 10 minutes, until cooked through. Stir occasionally.

2. Divide the lettuce evenly between four bowls. Add one-quarter of the beef mixture to each bowl and top with one-quarter of the tomatoes and cheese.

OPTION: Top with Creamy Avocado Dressing (page 139).

COMPLETE THE MEAL: Pair with your favorite vegetable side dish, such as steamed broccoli or sautéed red bell peppers, to get an adequate amount of carbohydrates.

NUTRITIONAL INFORMATION: Calories: 351; Total Fat: 18g; Protein: 35g; Carbohydrates: 14g; Sugars: 4g; Fiber: 6g; Sodium: 424mg

Sofrito Beef Tips

Carbs per serving: 6g

6 SERVINGS | **PREP TIME:** 5 minutes | **COOK TIME:** 30 minutes

For many people, beef stew is high on their list of comfort foods, but with so many potatoes and a salty broth, it's not the best for women with GDM. This flavorful twist on beef stew will satisfy your cravings and can be prepared in a fraction of the time it takes to make the traditional recipe.

1½ pounds stew beef chunks

½ head cauliflower

2 cups fresh or frozen broccoli florets

6 ounces *recaíto* cooking base (see page 72)

1. In a pressure cooker, place the beef on one side and the vegetables on the other. Pour in the *recaíto*.

2. Cook on the "Meat/Stew" setting.

3. When done cooking, mash the vegetables with a fork, breaking them down into a rice-like texture.

4. Divide the vegetables into six portions, and top each portion with one-sixth of the beef and sauce.

OPTION: You can also use a slow cooker. Cook the beef and vegetables on low for 8 hours.

COMPLETE THE MEAL: This meal is very low in carbohydrates, so consider pairing it with a large side salad or ½ cup corn.

NUTRITIONAL INFORMATION: Calories: 337; Total Fat: 18g; Protein: 32g; Carbohydrates: 6g; Sugars: 2; Fiber: 3g; Sodium: 294mg

Slow Cooker Ropa Vieja

Carbs per serving: 15g

---

4 SERVINGS | **PREP TIME:** 5 minutes | **COOK TIME:** 20 minutes

---

Ropa vieja is the mouthwatering Cuban version of pot roast. It's so good that you may never make your usual pot roast recipe again. Simply adding a red bell pepper changes the flavor profile. Instead of serving this dish with rice, the cauliflower will break apart and provide the "rice" for this meal.

½ small yellow onion

1 red bell pepper

1 (14-ounce) can no-salt-added diced tomatoes

1 teaspoon dried oregano

½ teaspoon salt

½ teaspoon smoked paprika

½ teaspoon garlic powder

1 pound chuck beef roast, trimmed of visible fat

1 head cauliflower

1. Cut the onion and bell pepper into ½-inch-thick slices.

2. Place the onion, bell pepper, diced tomatoes with their juices, oregano, salt, paprika, and garlic powder in a slow cooker, then add the beef.

3. Place the head of cauliflower on top of the beef, and cook on low for 8 hours.

4. When fully cooked, the cauliflower will fall apart when scooped.

COMPLETE THE MEAL: Serve alongside a generous portion of additional vegetables or a side dish, such as Mushroom and Cauliflower Rice Risotto (page 87).

NUTRITIONAL INFORMATION: Calories: 356; Total Fat: 18g; Protein: 35g; Carbohydrates: 15g; Sugars: 7g; Fiber: 5g; Sodium: 420mg

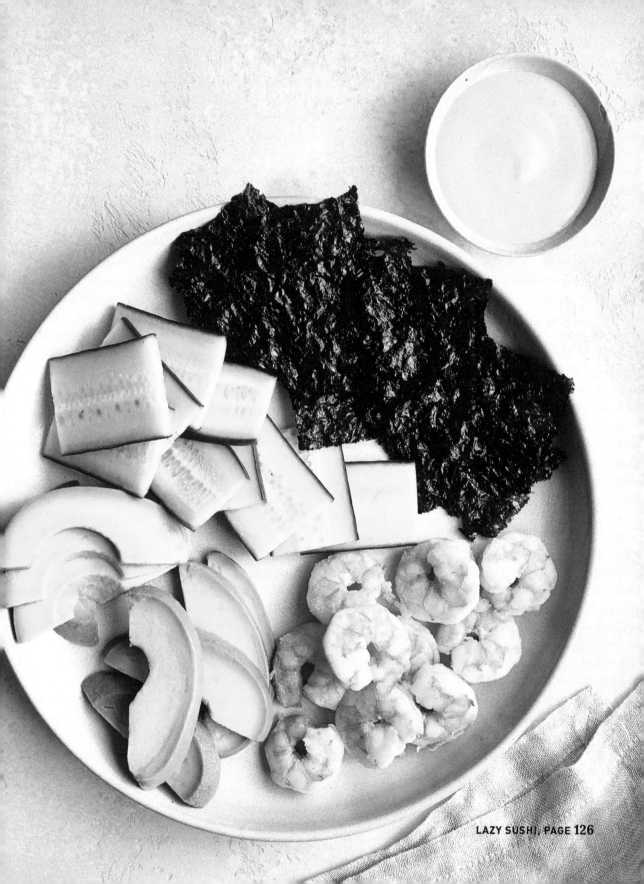

LAZY SUSHI, PAGE 126

Fish and Seafood

Lazy Sushi

Carbs per serving: 14g

2 SERVINGS | **PREP TIME:** 5 minutes | **COOK TIME:** 5 minutes

Sushi is a common pregnancy craving. I love Lazy Sushi because you get all of the sushi flavor without the carbs, plus you don't have to go through the trouble of cooking the rice and rolling the sushi. Since the shrimp is cooked, and it is a low-mercury fish, there aren't any safety concerns about eating this dish while pregnant.

20 medium fresh shrimp, peeled and deveined

1 teaspoon avocado oil

1 large cucumber

1 avocado

2 (4-gram) packages dried nori

¼ cup Spicy Asian-Style Sauce (page 144)

1. Heat a medium skillet over low heat.

2. In a large bowl, toss the shrimp with the oil, then place them into the skillet. Cook for 1 to 2 minutes on each side until they are pink and opaque. Set aside to cool.

3. Cut the cucumber into ¼-inch-thick planks about 2 inches long.

4. Cut the avocado into 10 slices.

5. Arrange half of the shrimp, cucumber, avocado, and nori on each of two plates, and serve with the sauce on the side.

INGREDIENT TIP: Be sure to use fresh shrimp rather than frozen, since frozen shrimp tend to have a lot of added salt. Use any remaining shrimp for Shrimp Stir-Fry (page 127).

COMPLETE THE MEAL: Accompany each serving with 1 cup shelled edamame to achieve a proper balance of carbohydrates, protein, and fat.

NUTRITIONAL INFORMATION: Calories: 266g; Total Fat: 19g; Protein: 15g; Carbohydrates: 14g; Sugars: 3g; Fiber: 7g; Sodium: 275mg

Shrimp Stir-Fry

Carbs per serving: 14g

4 SERVINGS | **PREP TIME:** 5 minutes | **COOK TIME:** 15 minutes

Stir-fry is always a great choice because it's an easy way to get in extra vegetables. Shrimp is one of the best sources of iodine, a mineral that many people are deficient in. Iodine helps both your and your baby's thyroid function and also assists with your baby's brain development. Seaweed is also rich in iodine, so fit in some nori whenever you can.

FOR THE SAUCE

½ cup water

2½ tablespoons low-sodium soy sauce

2 tablespoons honey

1 tablespoon rice vinegar

¼ teaspoon garlic powder

Pinch ground ginger

1 tablespoon cornstarch

FOR THE STIR-FRY

8 cups frozen vegetable stir-fry mix

2 tablespoons sesame oil

40 medium fresh shrimp, peeled and deveined

TO MAKE THE SAUCE

1. In a small saucepan, whisk together the water, soy sauce, honey, rice vinegar, garlic powder, and ginger. Add the cornstarch and whisk until fully incorporated.

2. Bring the sauce to a boil over medium heat. Boil for 1 minute to thicken. Remove the sauce from the heat and set aside.

TO MAKE THE STIR-FRY

1. Heat a large saucepan over medium-high heat. When hot, put the vegetable stir-fry mix into the pan, and cook for 7 to 10 minutes, stirring occasionally until the water completely evaporates.

2. Reduce the heat to medium-low, add the oil and shrimp, and stir. Cook for about 3 minutes, or until the shrimp are pink and opaque.

3. Add the sauce to the shrimp and vegetables and stir to coat. Cook for 2 minutes more.

COMPLETE THE MEAL: Enjoy 1 cup shelled edamame with each portion to achieve the proper balance of carbohydrates, protein, and fat.

NUTRITIONAL INFORMATION: Calories: 297; Total Fat: 17g; Protein: 24g; Carbohydrates: 14g; Sugars: 9g; Fiber: 2g; Sodium: 454mg

Fish Tacos

Carbs per serving: 30g

4 SERVINGS (2 TACOS = 1 SERVING) | **PREP TIME:** 5 minutes | **COOK TIME:** 10 minutes

Fish tacos are a fun, easy meal for the family, and they take little time to prepare. The bonus is that when made with cod, like these tacos are, they are also extremely nutritious. The tangy sauce adds a festive flavor to this perfectly balanced meal.

FOR THE TACOS

2 tablespoons extra-virgin olive oil

4 (6-ounce) cod fillets

8 (10-inch) yellow corn tortillas

2 cups packaged shredded cabbage

¼ cup chopped fresh cilantro

4 lime wedges

FOR THE SAUCE

½ cup plain low-fat Greek yogurt

⅓ cup low-fat mayonnaise

½ teaspoon garlic powder

½ teaspoon ground cumin

TO MAKE THE TACOS

1. Heat a medium skillet over medium-low heat. When hot, pour the oil into the skillet, then add the fish and cover. Cook for 4 minutes, then flip and cook for 4 minutes more.

2. Top each tortilla with one-eighth of the cabbage, sauce, cilantro, and fish. Finish each taco with a squeeze of lime.

TO MAKE THE SAUCE

In a small bowl, whisk together the yogurt, mayonnaise, garlic powder, and cumin.

COMPLETE THE MEAL: This recipe is balanced as it is, but any meal can always afford a side of vegetables. Try it with Cauliflower Steaks (page 82).

NUTRITIONAL INFORMATION: Calories: 373; Total Fat: 13g; Protein: 36g; Carbohydrates: 30g; Sugars: 4g; Fiber: 4g; Sodium: 342mg

Lemon Butter Cod with Asparagus

Carbs per serving: 20g

4 SERVINGS | **PREP TIME:** 5 minutes | **COOK TIME:** 15 minutes

A rich, bright lemon butter sauce gives a whole new flavor profile to this simple fish and vegetable pairing. One fillet of cod contains about 75 percent of your recommended daily iodine and over twice as much potassium as a banana. Potassium helps maintain normal blood pressure and prevents swelling, which is extremely helpful as pregnancy progresses.

½ cup uncooked brown rice or quinoa

4 (4-ounce) cod fillets

¼ teaspoon salt

¼ teaspoon freshly ground black pepper

¼ teaspoon garlic powder

24 asparagus spears

2 tablespoons unsalted butter

1 tablespoon freshly squeezed lemon juice

1. Cook the rice according to the package instructions.

2. Meanwhile, season both sides of the cod fillets with the salt, pepper, and garlic powder.

3. Cut the bottom 1½ inches from the asparagus.

4. Heat a large skillet over medium-low heat. When hot, melt the butter in the skillet, then arrange the cod and asparagus in a single layer.

5. Cover and cook for 8 minutes.

6. Divide the rice, fish, and asparagus into four equal portions. Drizzle with the lemon juice to finish.

COMPLETE THE MEAL: This dish pairs well with Mushroom and Cauliflower Rice Risotto (page 87) or Cauliflower Leek Soup (page 60) for added carbohydrates.

NUTRITIONAL INFORMATION: Calories: 230; Total Fat: 8g; Protein: 22g; Carbohydrates: 20g; Sugars: 2g; Fiber: 5g; Sodium: 274mg

Creamy Cod with Asparagus

Carbs per serving: 23g

4 SERVINGS | **PREP TIME:** 5 minutes | **COOK TIME:** 15 minutes

Cod is a low-mercury fish that allows pregnant women to get the full benefits of seafood, including high levels of vitamin D and omega-3 fatty acids. The FDA encourages pregnant women to eat two or three servings of low-mercury fish per week, and it names cod, salmon, shrimp, and canned light tuna among the best choices for moms-to-be.

½ cup uncooked brown rice or quinoa

4 (4-ounce) cod fillets

¼ teaspoon salt

¼ teaspoon freshly ground black pepper

½ teaspoon garlic powder, divided

24 asparagus spears

Avocado oil cooking spray

1 cup half-and-half

1. Cook the rice according to the package instructions.

2. Meanwhile, season both sides of the cod fillets with the salt, pepper, and ¼ teaspoon of garlic powder.

3. Cut the bottom 1½ inches from the asparagus.

4. Heat a large pan over medium-low heat. When hot, coat the cooking surface with cooking spray, and arrange the cod and asparagus in a single layer.

5. Cover and cook for 8 minutes.

6. Add the half-and-half and the remaining ¼ teaspoon of garlic powder and stir. Increase the heat to high and simmer for 2 minutes.

7. Divide the rice, cod, and asparagus into four equal portions.

COMPLETE THE MEAL: This recipe pairs well with Mushroom and Cauliflower Rice Risotto (page 87), or you can simply add an additional ¼ cup cooked brown rice or quinoa to each portion for a more filling meal.

NUTRITIONAL INFORMATION: Calories: 257; Total Fat: 8g; Protein: 25g; Carbohydrates: 23g; Sugars: 4g; Fiber: 5g; Sodium: 411mg

Catfish with Corn and Pepper Relish

Carbs per serving: 27g

---

4 SERVINGS | **PREP TIME:** 10 minutes | **COOK TIME:** 10 minutes

---

Catfish is a low-mercury fish that is rich in omega-3 fatty acids. Most people do not get enough omega-3s in their diet. Sufficient omega-3s can lower anxiety and improve eye health. They also promote healthy brain development in babies, so try to incorporate seafood—the perfect natural source of omega-3s—into your diet two or three times per week.

---

3 tablespoons extra-virgin olive oil, divided

4 (5-ounce) catfish fillets

¼ teaspoon salt

¼ teaspoon freshly ground black pepper

1 (15-ounce) can low-sodium black beans, drained and rinsed

1 cup frozen corn

1 medium red bell pepper, diced

1 tablespoon apple cider vinegar

3 tablespoons chopped scallions

1. Use 1½ tablespoons of oil to coat both sides of the catfish fillets, then season the fillets with the salt and pepper.

2. Heat a small saucepan over medium-high heat. Put the remaining 1½ tablespoons of oil, beans, corn, bell pepper, and vinegar in the pan and stir. Cover and cook for 5 minutes.

3. Place the catfish fillets on top of the relish mixture and cover. Cook for 5 to 7 minutes.

4. Serve each catfish fillet with one-quarter of the relish and top with the scallions.

> OPTION: Substitute 2 tablespoons of freshly squeezed lemon juice for the vinegar.

NUTRITIONAL INFORMATION: Calories: 409; Total Fat: 21g; Protein: 28g; Carbohydrates: 27g; Sugars: 4g; Fiber: 6g; Sodium: 341mg

Lemon Pepper Salmon

Carbs per serving: 10g

4 SERVINGS | **PREP TIME:** 5 minutes | **COOK TIME:** 20 minutes, plus 5 minutes to rest

The wonderful thing about salmon is that it doesn't need a lot of dressing up. The rich flavor and firm texture can practically stand alone. This recipe uses just a splash of fresh lemon juice and freshly ground black pepper to highlight the flavor of the salmon. Brussels sprouts round out the dish.

Avocado oil cooking spray

20 Brussels sprouts, halved lengthwise

4 (4-ounce) skinless salmon fillets

½ teaspoon garlic powder

½ teaspoon freshly ground black pepper

¼ teaspoon salt

2 teaspoons freshly squeezed lemon juice

1. Heat a large skillet over medium-low heat. When hot, coat the cooking surface with cooking spray, and put the Brussels sprouts cut-side down in the skillet. Cover and cook for 5 minutes.

2. Meanwhile, season both sides of the salmon with the garlic powder, pepper, and salt.

3. Flip the Brussels sprouts, and move them to one side of the skillet. Add the salmon and cook, uncovered, for 4 to 6 minutes.

4. Check the Brussels sprouts. When they are tender, remove them from the skillet and set them aside.

5. Flip the salmon fillets. Cook for 4 to 6 more minutes, or until the salmon is opaque and flakes easily with a fork. Remove the salmon from the skillet, and let it rest for 5 minutes.

6. Divide the Brussels sprouts into four equal portions and add 1 salmon fillet to each portion. Sprinkle the lemon juice on top and serve.

COMPLETE THE MEAL: This dish is not meant to be consumed alone because it is low in calories, fat, and carbohydrates. Consider pairing it with Italian Zucchini Boats (page 93) or Cauliflower Leek Soup (page 60).

NUTRITIONAL INFORMATION: Calories: 193; Total Fat: 7g; Protein: 25g; Carbohydrates: 10g; Sugars: 2g; Fiber: 4g; Sodium: 222mg

Salmon with Brussels Sprouts

Carbs per serving: 9g

4 SERVINGS | **PREP TIME:** 5 minutes | **COOK TIME:** 20 minutes

Brussels sprouts go so well with salmon that I'm including two recipes that pair these ingredients. In this dish, two superfoods come together to provide a meal jam-packed with nutrients.

2 tablespoons unsalted butter, divided

20 Brussels sprouts, halved lengthwise

4 (4-ounce) skinless salmon fillets

½ teaspoon salt

¼ teaspoon garlic powder

1. Heat a medium skillet over medium-low heat. When hot, melt 1 tablespoon of butter in the skillet, then add the Brussels sprouts cut-side down. Cook for 10 minutes.

2. Season both sides of the salmon fillets with the salt and garlic powder.

3. Heat another medium skillet over medium-low heat. When hot, melt the remaining 1 tablespoon of butter in the skillet, then add the salmon. Cover and cook for 6 to 8 minutes, or until the salmon is opaque and flakes easily with a fork.

4. Meanwhile, flip the Brussels sprouts and cover. Cook for 10 minutes or until tender.

5. Divide the Brussels sprouts into four equal portions and add 1 salmon fillet to each portion.

COMPLETE THE MEAL: Serve with ½ cup cooked brown rice or quinoa, seasoned as desired.

NUTRITIONAL INFORMATION: Calories: 243; Total Fat: 13g; Protein: 25g; Carbohydrates: 9g; Sugars: 2g; Fiber: 4g; Sodium: 222mg

Avo-Tuna with Croutons

Carbs per serving: 19g

---

3 SERVINGS (2 AVOCADO HALVES, FILLED = 1 SERVING) | **PREP TIME:** 10 minutes

---

This easy lunch will keep you going on the days when your time is at a premium. With hardly any prep required, you can throw this recipe together between sips of decaf coffee before you head out the door in the morning. With the addition of a small piece of whole fruit, you'll have a perfectly balanced lunch.

---

2 (5-ounce) cans chunk-light tuna, drained

2 tablespoons low-fat mayonnaise

½ teaspoon freshly ground black pepper

3 avocados, halved and pitted

6 tablespoons packaged croutons

1. In a medium bowl, combine the tuna, mayonnaise, and pepper, and mix well.

2. Top the avocados with the tuna mixture and croutons.

INGREDIENT TIP: Be sure to purchase only chunk-light tuna, which is lower in mercury than albacore tuna. Safe Catch is a good brand that tests its fish and meets the low-mercury standard for pregnant women.

NUTRITIONAL INFORMATION: Calories: 428; Total Fat: 29g; Protein: 28g; Carbohydrates: 19g; Sugars: 1g; Fiber: 12g; Sodium: 167mg

Tuna Casserole

Carbs per serving: 11g

---

4 SERVINGS | **PREP TIME:** 10 minutes | **COOK TIME:** 40 minutes

---

Tuna noodle casserole is one of those yummy comfort foods that you realize as an adult is full of ingredients that are not particularly conducive to good health. This adaptation replaces high-carbohydrate pasta with zucchini noodles and the overly rich béchamel with an almond milk version. And guess what? It's still topped with plenty of melted Cheddar cheese. Enjoy!

Avocado oil cooking spray

1 medium yellow onion, diced

2 tablespoons whole-wheat flour

2 cups low-sodium chicken broth

1 cup unsweetened almond milk

1 cup fresh or frozen broccoli florets

1 (10-ounce) package zucchini noodles

2 (5-ounce) cans chunk-light tuna, drained

1 cup shredded Cheddar cheese

1. Preheat the oven to 375°F.

2. Heat a medium skillet over medium heat. When hot, coat the cooking surface with cooking spray. Put the onion into the skillet and cook for 3 minutes.

3. Add the flour and stir. Cook for 2 minutes, stirring once.

4. Add the broth slowly, then the almond milk, stirring constantly.

5. Increase the heat to high. Once the mixture comes to a boil, add the broccoli and noodles. Reduce the heat to medium and cook for 5 to 7 minutes. The mixture will thicken.

6. Add the tuna and stir.

7. Transfer the mixture to an 8-by-8-inch casserole dish and top with the cheese.

8. Cover with foil and bake for 20 minutes.

9. Uncover and broil for 2 minutes.

COMPLETE THE MEAL: Since this meal is low in calories and carbohydrates, pair it with a vegetable dish, such as Italian Zucchini Boats (page 93) or a large side salad.

NUTRITIONAL INFORMATION: Calories: 269; Total Fat: 12g; Protein: 29g; Carbohydrates: 11g; Sugars: 3g; Fiber: 3g; Sodium: 351mg

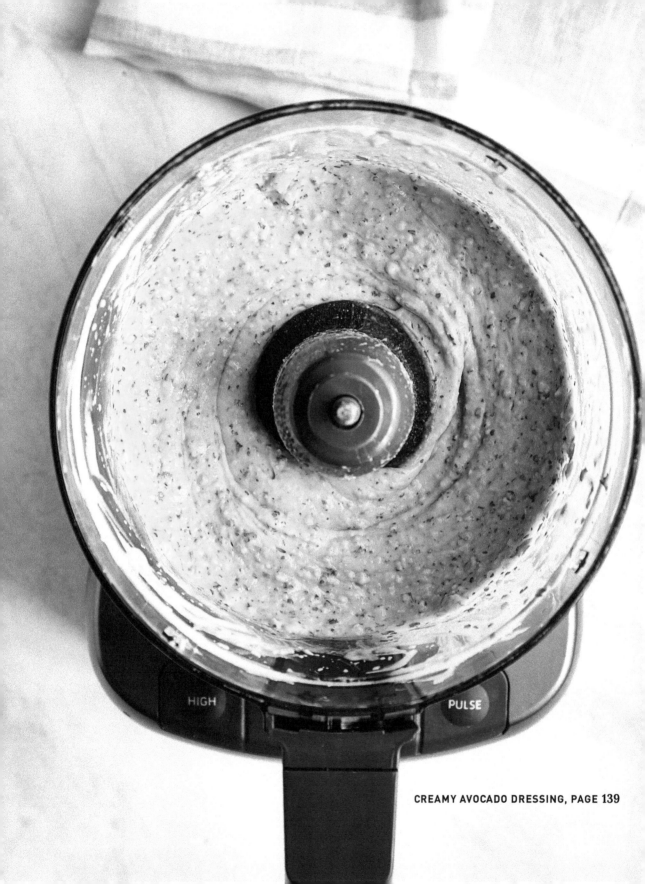

HIGH PULSE

CREAMY AVOCADO DRESSING, PAGE 139

Staples

Lemon Cream Sauce

Carbs per serving: 1g

MAKES 2 CUPS (¼ CUP = 1 SERVING) | **PREP TIME:** 5 minutes | **COOK TIME:** 5 minutes

This is an elegant sauce that guests will think you painstakingly perfected. Little will they know it took you less than 10 minutes to make. It pairs beautifully with chicken and white fish, but it is one recipe in this book that should not be made too far ahead. Whip this up right before you plan to use it, ideally when your chicken or fish is in the last 3 minutes of cooking.

1 cup half-and-half

2 tablespoons shredded Parmesan cheese

1 tablespoon unsalted butter

1 teaspoon freshly squeezed lemon juice

¼ teaspoon garlic powder

1. Heat a small saucepan over medium-low heat.

2. Put the half-and-half, cheese, butter, lemon juice, and garlic powder into the pan and stir. Let the sauce heat through before serving.

STORAGE TIP: Store in a closed container in the refrigerator for up to 1 day.

NUTRITIONAL INFORMATION: Calories: 53; Total Fat: 5g; Protein: 2g; Carbohydrates: 1g; Sugars: 0g; Fiber: 0g; Sodium: 39mg

Creamy Avocado Dressing

Carbs per serving: 4g

MAKES 1 CUP (¼ CUP = 1 SERVING) | **PREP TIME:** 5 minutes

Avocado dressing is a versatile dressing that is great on salad greens and raw or cooked vegetables. It's also great with Latin-inspired recipes. It is the perfect substitute for ranch because it gives you that creamy texture and tangy zip you love. If you like, you can add water to make it a thinner consistency without diluting the flavor.

½ cup plain low-fat Greek yogurt

1 large avocado, peeled and pitted

¾ cup fresh cilantro, loosely packed

2 teaspoons freshly squeezed lime juice

1 tablespoon water

⅛ teaspoon garlic powder

Pinch salt

Put the yogurt, avocado, cilantro, lime juice, water, garlic powder, and salt into a blender and blend well.

OPTION: Fresh lime juice gives a bright pop, but bottled juice works, too.

STORAGE TIP: Store this dressing in a closed container in the refrigerator for up to 5 days or freeze for up to 2 months if you won't use it immediately. The sauce may brown, but it will still be good.

NUTRITIONAL INFORMATION: Calories: 93; Total Fat: 7g; Protein: 4g; Carbohydrates: 5g; Sugars: 1g; Fiber: 2g; Sodium: 53mg

Creamy Dill Dressing

Carbs per serving: 3g

MAKES ⅔ CUP (2½ TABLESPOONS = 1 SERVING) | **PREP TIME:** 5 minutes

---

The flavor of fresh dill is so unique that it makes any dish special. This dressing is equally delicious over raw spring vegetables or a salmon fillet. It pairs well with a delicate cucumber salad, but it will also hold up to more hearty dishes, like roasted vegetables. In the end, you'll love this dressing so much, you'll want to put it on everything.

½ cup plain low-fat Greek yogurt

2 tablespoons low-fat mayonnaise

1 teaspoon chopped fresh dill

1 teaspoon freshly squeezed lemon juice

¼ teaspoon garlic powder

¼ teaspoon salt

In a small bowl, whisk together the yogurt, mayonnaise, dill, lemon juice, garlic powder, and salt.

STORAGE TIP: Store in a closed container in the refrigerator for up to 2 weeks.

INGREDIENT TIP: Freeze leftover dill until you're ready to use it. Dried dill lacks the flavor of fresh dill.

NUTRITIONAL INFORMATION: Calories: 35; Total Fat: 1g; Protein: 3g; Carbohydrates: 3g; Sugars: 2g; Fiber: 0g; Sodium: 178mg

Creamy Lemon Tahini Dressing

Carbs per serving: 10g

MAKES 1 CUP (2 TABLESPOONS = 1 SERVING) | **PREP TIME:** 5 minutes

Tahini is made from sesame seeds. It is used in many Middle Eastern dishes and is primarily known as one of the main ingredients in hummus. The sesame flavor in this dressing is complemented by the honey and lemon. This dressing is the perfect balance of savory, sweet, and tangy. It pairs nicely with chicken and salads.

¾ cup unsalted tahini

½ cup water

⅓ cup freshly squeezed lemon juice

3 tablespoons honey

½ teaspoon salt

In a medium bowl, whisk together the tahini, water, lemon juice, honey, and salt. If it looks like it's not combining, mix a bit more vigorously, and it will come together.

STORAGE TIP: Store in a closed container in the refrigerator for up to 2 weeks. Shake well before using again.

NUTRITIONAL INFORMATION: Calories: 170; Total Fat: 13g; Protein: 5g; Carbohydrates: 10g; Sugars: 8g; Fiber: 3g; Sodium: 150mg

Roasted Red Pepper Spread

Carbs per serving: 5g

MAKES 1¼ CUPS (2 TABLESPOONS = 1 SERVING) | **PREP TIME:** 5 minutes

This spread is sure to spice up your life and give your palate something new to sing about. Try it on avocado toast or eggs or use it as a salsa replacement. Make it ahead of time and keep it in the refrigerator. It's so good, you'll always want to have some on hand.

---

1 (16-ounce) jar roasted red bell peppers

1 cup canned low-sodium chickpeas, drained and rinsed

½ small jalapeño pepper, seeded and stemmed

2 tablespoons extra-virgin olive oil

2 tablespoons water

1 to 2 teaspoons freshly squeezed lime juice

½ teaspoon salt

¼ teaspoon garlic powder

¼ teaspoon ground cumin

⅛ teaspoon freshly ground black pepper

Put the bell peppers, chickpeas, jalapeño pepper, oil, water, lime juice, salt, garlic powder, cumin, and black pepper into a food processor or blender and blend until smooth. The sauce will have texture, but it shouldn't be chunky.

OPTION: Add 2 to 3 tablespoons of unsalted tahini for a twist on roasted red pepper hummus.

STORAGE TIP: Store in a closed container in the refrigerator for up to 1 week.

NUTRITIONAL INFORMATION: Calories: 53; Total Fat: 3g; Protein: 1g; Carbohydrates: 5g; Sugars: 2g; Fiber: 2g; Sodium: 139mg

Garlic Mayo-Ketchup

Carbs per serving: 3g

MAKES 1 CUP (2 TABLESPOONS = 1 SERVING) | **PREP TIME:** 5 minutes

---

This addictive sauce is a staple in Puerto Rico. You can use it to replace your regular plain mayonnaise or ketchup. The garlic flavor gives it an extra kick. Add ½ teaspoon freshly ground black pepper to bump up the flavor even more.

½ cup low-fat mayonnaise

6 tablespoons no-salt-added, no-sugar-added ketchup

1 teaspoon garlic powder

In a small bowl, mix the mayonnaise, ketchup, and garlic powder together until well combined.

STORAGE TIP: Store in a closed container in the refrigerator for up to 2 weeks.

NUTRITIONAL INFORMATION: Calories: 44; Total Fat: 3g; Protein: 0g; Carbohydrates: 3g; Sugars: 1g; Fiber: 0g; Sodium: 169mg

GLUTEN-FREE, VEGETARIAN, DAIRY-FREE, NUT-FREE,
5-INGREDIENT, 30 MINUTES OR LESS, NO COOK

Spicy Asian-Style Sauce

Carbs per serving: 2g

MAKES ½ CUP (2 TABLESPOONS = 1 SERVING) | **PREP TIME:** 5 minutes

You're probably familiar with a version of this sauce if you've ever had a spicy tuna roll or other spicy sushi. The hot sauce provides more flavor than heat, and the spice is barely noticeable when eaten with a meal. Feel free to increase the amount of hot sauce if you're a fan of spicy food.

⅓ cup low-fat mayonnaise

2 teaspoons rice vinegar

1 to 2 teaspoons hot sauce, to your liking

1 teaspoon sesame oil

In a small bowl, whisk together the mayonnaise, rice vinegar, hot sauce, and sesame oil.

STORAGE TIP: Store in a closed container in the refrigerator for up to 2 weeks.

NUTRITIONAL INFORMATION: Calories: 55; Total Fat: 5g; Protein: 0g; Carbohydrates: 2g; Sugars: 1g; Fiber: 0g; Sodium: 191mg

Thai-Style Peanut Sauce

Carbs per serving: 8g

MAKES ⅔ CUP (2½ TABLESPOONS = 1 SERVING) | **PREP TIME:** 10 minutes

Homemade Thai-style food is easy with this flavorful sauce. It will appear thick when cold but will melt when it touches hot food. You can also thin the consistency with water, if you'd like. If you can't find fresh ginger, feel free to use a pinch of ground ginger instead.

½ cup natural peanut butter

4 teaspoons sesame oil

2 tablespoons rice vinegar

1 teaspoon chopped peeled fresh ginger or pinch ground ginger

2 to 4 teaspoons freshly squeezed lime juice, to your liking

2 to 2½ teaspoons hot sauce (optional)

1 teaspoon low-sodium soy sauce

1 teaspoon honey

1. In a small bowl, whisk together the peanut butter, sesame oil, and rice vinegar. The peanut butter will become more pliable as you whisk.

2. Whisk in the ginger.

3. Whisk in the lime juice, hot sauce (if using), soy sauce, and honey.

> **STORAGE TIP:** Store in a closed container in the refrigerator for up to 2 weeks. Bring to room temperature and stir well before using again.

NUTRITIONAL INFORMATION: Calories: 207; Total Fat: 17g; Protein: 8g; Carbohydrates: 8g; Sugars: 3g; Fiber: 3g; Sodium: 115mg

The Dirty Dozen and the Clean Fifteen™

A nonprofit environmental watchdog organization called Environmental Working Group looks at data supplied by the U.S. Department of Agriculture and the Food and Drug Administration about pesticide residues. Each year, it compiles a list of the best and worst pesticide loads found in commercial crops. You can use these lists to decide which fruits and vegetables to buy organic to minimize your exposure to pesticides and which produce is considered safe enough to buy conventionally. Safe to buy does not mean pesticide-free, though, so wash these fruits and vegetables thoroughly. The list is updated annually, and you can find it online at EWG.org/FoodNews.

DIRTY DOZEN™

1. Strawberries
2. Spinach
3. Kale
4. Nectarines
5. Apples
6. Grapes
7. Peaches
8. Cherries
9. Pears
10. Tomatoes
11. Celery
12. Potatoes

Additionally, nearly three-quarters of hot pepper samples contained pesticide residues.

CLEAN FIFTEEN™

1. Avocados
2. Sweet corn
3. Pineapples
4. Sweet peas (frozen)
5. Onions
6. Papayas
7. Eggplants
8. Asparagus
9. Kiwis
10. Cabbages
11. Cauliflower
12. Cantaloupes
13. Broccoli
14. Mushrooms
15. Honeydew melons

Measurement Conversions

VOLUME EQUIVALENTS (LIQUID)

U.S. STANDARD	U.S. STANDARD (OUNCES)	METRIC (APPROXIMATE)
2 tablespoons	1 fl. oz.	30 mL
¼ cup	2 fl. oz.	60 mL
½ cup	4 fl. oz.	120 mL
1 cup	8 fl. oz.	240 mL
1½ cups	12 fl. oz.	355 mL
2 cups or 1 pint	16 fl. oz.	475 mL
4 cups or 1 quart	32 fl. oz.	1 L
1 gallon	128 fl. oz.	4 L

VOLUME EQUIVALENTS (DRY)

U.S. STANDARD	METRIC (APPROXIMATE)
⅛ teaspoon	0.5 mL
¼ teaspoon	1 mL
½ teaspoon	2 mL
¾ teaspoon	4 mL
1 teaspoon	5 mL
1 tablespoon	15 mL
¼ cup	59 mL
⅓ cup	79 mL
½ cup	118 mL
⅔ cup	156 mL
¾ cup	177 mL
1 cup	235 mL
2 cups or 1 pint	475 mL
3 cups	700 mL
4 cups or 1 quart	1 L

OVEN TEMPERATURES

FAHRENHEIT (F)	CELSIUS (C) (APPROXIMATE)
250°F	120°C
300°F	150°C
325°F	165°C
350°F	180°C
375°F	190°C
400°F	200°C
425°F	220°C
450°F	230°C

WEIGHT EQUIVALENTS

U.S. STANDARD	METRIC (APPROXIMATE)
½ ounce	15 g
1 ounce	30 g
2 ounces	60 g
4 ounces	115 g
8 ounces	225 g
12 ounces	340 g
16 ounces or 1 pound	455 g

Glycemic Index and Glycemic Load Food List

The following is a list of the glycemic index and glycemic load of many common foods. Foods are ranked between 0 and 100 based on how they affect one's blood glucose level. The best choices are low glycemic, which have a rating of 55 or less, and medium glycemic, which have a rating of 56 to 69.

Remember that it is more important to pay attention to the glycemic load of a food, that is, the amount of carbohydrates it contains per serving. The best choices have low (less than 10) or moderate (between 10 and 20) loads.

GLYCEMIC INDEX AND GLYCEMIC LOAD OF COMMON FOODS

Food	Glycemic Index	Serving Size (grams)	Glycemic Load (per serving)
BAKERY PRODUCTS			
Bagel, white	72	70	25
Baguette, white	95	30	15
Barley bread	34	30	7
Corn tortilla	52	50	12
Croissant	67	57	17
Doughnut	76	47	17
Pita bread	68	30	10
Sourdough rye	48	30	6
Soya and linseed bread	36	30	3
Sponge cake	46	63	17
Wheat tortilla	30	50	8
White-wheat-flour bread	71	30	10
Whole-wheat bread	71	30	9
BEVERAGES			
Apple juice, unsweetened	44	250 mL	30
Coca-Cola	63	250 mL	16
Gatorade	78	250 mL	12
Lucozade	95	250 mL	40
Orange juice, unsweetened	50	250 mL	12
Tomato juice, canned	38	250 mL	4

Food	Glycemic Index	Serving Size (grams)	Glycemic Load (per serving)
BREAKFAST CEREALS			
All-Bran	55	30	12
Coco Pops	77	30	20
Cornflakes	93	30	23
Muesli	66	30	16
Oatmeal	55	50	13
Special K	69	30	14
DAIRY			
Ice cream, regular	57	50	6
Milk, full fat	41	250 mL	5
Milk, skim	32	250 mL	4
Reduced-fat yogurt with fruit	33	200	11
FRUITS			
Apple	39	120	6
Banana, ripe	62	120	16
Cherries	22	120	3
Dates, dried	42	60	18
Grapefruit	25	120	3
Grapes	59	120	11
Mango	41	120	8
Orange	40	120	4
Peach	42	120	5
Pear	38	120	4
Pineapple	51	120	8
Raisins	64	60	28
Strawberries	40	120	1
Watermelon	72	120	4

Food	Glycemic Index	Serving Size (grams)	Glycemic Load (per serving)
GRAINS			
Brown rice	50	150	16
Buckwheat	45	150	13
Bulgur	30	50	11
Corn on the cob	60	150	20
Couscous	65	150	9
Fettucini	32	180	15
Gnocchi	68	180	33
Macaroni	47	180	23
Quinoa	53	150	13
Spaghetti, white	46	180	22
Spaghetti, whole wheat	42	180	26
Vermicelli	35	180	16
White rice	89	150	43
LEGUMES			
Baked beans	40	150	6
Black beans	30	150	7
Butter beans	36	150	8
Chickpeas	10	150	3
Kidney beans	29	150	7
Lentils	29	150	5
Navy beans	31	150	9
Soybeans	50	150	1

Food	Glycemic Index	Serving Size (grams)	Glycemic Load (per serving)
SNACK FOODS			
Cashews, salted	27	50	3
Corn chips, salted	42	50	11
Fruit Roll-Ups	99	30	24
Graham crackers	74	25	14
Honey	61	25	12
Hummus	6	30	0
M&M's, peanut	33	30	6
Microwave popcorn, plain	55	20	6
Muesli bar	61	30	13
Nutella	33	20	4
Peanuts	7	50	0
Potato chips	51	50	12
Pretzels	83	30	16
Rice cakes	82	25	17
Rye crisps	64	25	11
Shortbread	64	25	10
Vanilla wafers	77	25	14
VEGETABLES			
Beetroot	64	80	4
Carrot	35	80	2
Green peas	51	80	4
Parsnip	52	80	4
Sweet potato	70	150	22
White potato, boiled	81	150	22
Yam	54	150	20

Sources: Harvard Health Publications (http://www.health.harvard.edu/healthy-eating/glycemic_index_and_glycemic_load_for_100_foods) and Mendosa.com (http://www.mendosa.com/gilists.htm).

Carbohydrate and Calorie Values

Understanding the carbohydrate and calorie content of common foods can help you plan your meals. These values are derived from NutritionData.com, which is a useful site for calculating nutritional information.

BREADS, CEREALS & PASTAS

Each of the serving sizes listed below offers 15g carbs:

- » Barley, cooked (⅓ cup); 70 cals
- » Bread, white or whole wheat, pumpernickel, rye (1 slice or 1 ounce); 65 cals
- » Bun, hamburger/hot dog (½ bun or 1 ounce), 80 cals
- » Couscous, cooked (⅓ cup); 60 cals
- » Crackers, Saltine or round butter (4 to 6); 70 cals
- » English muffin (½); 65 cals
- » Melba toast (4 slices); 60 cals
- » Oyster crackers (20); 100 cals
- » Pasta, cooked (⅓ cup); 75 cals
- » Quinoa, cooked (½ cup), 70 cals
- » Rice, white or brown, cooked (⅓ cup); 70 cals
- » Tortilla, corn or flour (6 inches across); 60 cals

STARCHY VEGETABLES

Each of the serving sizes listed below offers 15g carbs:

- » Butternut squash, cooked (¾ cup); 75 cals
- » Corn (½ cup); 65 cals
- » Potato, baked (1 small or ¼ large or 3 ounces); 57 cals
- » Pumpkin, cooked (1 cup, cubed); 50 cals
- » Sweet potato (½ cup); 54 cals

BEANS & LENTILS

Each of the serving sizes listed below offers 12–15g carbs:

- » Baked beans (¼ cup); 60 cals
- » Black beans, cooked (¼ cup); 70 cals
- » Chickpeas, cooked (¼ cup); 90 cals
- » Hummus (⅓ cup); 135 cals
- » Kidney beans, cooked (¼ cup); 70 cals
- » Lentils, cooked (½ cup); 64 cals
- » Lima beans, cooked (¼ cup); 64 cals
- » Navy beans, cooked (¼ cup); 80 cals
- » Peas, black-eyed, split, cooked (½ cup); 57 cals
- » Pinto beans, cooked (¼ cup); 80 cals
- » White beans, cooked (¼ cup); 80 cals
- » Refried beans (½ cup); 92 cals

NONSTARCHY VEGETABLES

Each of the serving sizes listed below offers 15g carbs:

- » Beets, cooked (1 cup); 74 cals
- » Broccoli, cooked (1 cup chopped); 44 cals
- » Brussels sprouts, cooked (1 cup); 56 cals
- » Cabbage, raw (2 cups); 56 cals
- » Carrots, (1 cup); 70 cals
- » Cauliflower, raw (3 cups); 75 cals
- » Celery, raw (5 cups, chopped); 80 cals
- » Chard, raw (15 cups); 105 cals
- » Cucumber, raw (5 cups); 80 cals
- » Eggplant, raw (3 cups); 60 cals
- » Green beans, raw (2 cups); 70 cals
- » Kale, raw (2 cups); 66 cals
- » Okra, cooked (3 cups); 54 cals
- » Radishes, raw (3 cups); 57 cals
- » Romaine lettuce, shredded (6 cups); 48 cals
- » Spinach, raw (15 cups); 105 cals
- » Tomatoes, raw (2 cups); 54 cals
- » Zucchini, raw (3 cups); 60 cals

FRUIT

Each of the serving sizes listed below offers 15g carbs:

- » Apple (¾ cup, chopped); 60 cals
- » Apricots, raw (¾ cup); 65 cals
- » Banana (½ cup); 67 cals
- » Blueberries (¾ cup); 63 cals
- » Cantaloupe (1 cup, cubed); 60 cals
- » Cherries (12); 60 cals
- » Grapefruit, large (½); 52 cals
- » Grapes (1 cup); 62 cals
- » Kiwi (1); 56 cals
- » Mango (½ cup); 53 cals
- » Orange (1 small); 65 cals
- » Papaya (1 cup, cubed); 55 cals
- » Peach (1 medium); 59 cals
- » Pear (½ large); 66 cals
- » Pineapple (¾ cup); 63 cals
- » Plum (2 small); 60 cals
- » Raspberries (1 cup); 64 cals
- » Strawberries (1 cup, sliced), 53 cals
- » Watermelon (1¼ cups, cubed), 57 cals

DAIRY

Each of the serving sizes listed below offers 12–15g carbs:

- » Low-fat plain yogurt (⅔ cup); 100 cals
- » Milk, 2% (1 cup); 138 cals

References

American Diabetes Association. "What is Gestational Diabetes?" Updated March 21, 2017. https://www.diabetes.org/diabetes/gestational-diabetes.

Arnold, Greg. "Magnesium Benefits Blood Sugar Control during Pregnancy." Natural Research Institute. January 5, 2016. http://www.naturalhealthresearch.org/magnesium-benefits-blood-sugar-control-during-pregnancy-directors-choice-2/.

California Diabetes and Pregnancy Program. "California MyPlate for Gestational Diabetes." California Department of Public Health, 2018. https://www.cdph.ca.gov/Programs/CFH/DMCAH/CDPH%20Document%20Library/NUPA/MyPlate-Handout-GestationalDiabetes.pdf.

DeSisto, Carla L., Shin Y. Kim, and Andrea Sharma. "Prevalence Estimates of Gestational Diabetes Mellitus in the United States, Pregnancy Risk Assessment Monitoring System (PRAMS) 2007-2010," *Preventing Chronic Disease* 11, 130415 (June 19, 2014). http://dx.doi.org/10.5888/pcd11.130415.

Herath, Himali, Rasika Herath, and Rajitha Wickremasinghe. "Gestational Diabetes Mellitus and Risk of Type 2 Diabetes 10 Years after the Index Pregnancy in Sri Lankan Women: A Community Based Retrospective," *PLOS One* 12, no. 6 (June 23, 2017): e0179647. https://doi.org/10.1371/journal.pone.0179647.

Hernandez, Teri L., and Jennie Brand-Miller. "Nutrition Therapy in Gestational Diabetes Mellitus: Time to Move Forward," *Diabetes Care* 41, no. 7 (July 2018): 1343–45. https://doi.org/10.2337/dci18-0014.

Kim, Catherine, Diana K. Berger, and Shadi Chamany. "Recurrence of Gestational Diabetes Mellitus: A Systematic Review," *Diabetes Care* 30, no. 5 (May 2007): 1314–19. https://doi.org/10.2337/dc06-2517.

Mirghani, H. M., D. S. Weerasinghe, M. Ezimokhai, and J. R. Smith. "The Effect of Maternal Fasting on the Fetal Biophysics Profile." *International Journal of Gynaecology and Obstetrics* 81, no. 1 (April 2003): 17–21. http://www.fda.gov/media/117402/download.

Moses, Robert G., Megan Barker, Meagan Winter, Peter Petocz, and Jennie Brand-Miller. "Can a Low-Glycemic Index Diet Reduce the Need for Insulin in Gestational Diabetes Mellitus: A Randomized Trial." *Diabetes Care* 32, no. 6 (June 2009): 996–1000. https://doi.org/10.2337/dc09-0007.

National Center for Chronic Disease Prevention and Health Promotion. "Get the Facts: Sodium and the Dietary Guidelines." Centers for Disease Control and Prevention, 2017. https://www.cdc.gov/salt/pdfs/sodium_dietary_guidelines.pdf.

Pistollato, Francesca, Sandra Sumalla Cano, Iñaki Elio, Manuel Masias Vergara, Francesca Giampieri, and Maurizio Battino. "Plant-Based and Plant-Rich Diet Patterns during Gestation: Effects and Possible Shortcomings." *Advances in Nutrition* 6, no. 5 (September 2015): 581–91. https://doi.org/10.3945/an.115.009126.

Tobias, Dierdre K., Frank B. Hu, John P. Forman, Jorge Chavarro, and Cuilin Zhang. "Increased Risk of Hypertension after Gestational Diabetes Mellitus: Findings from a Large Prospective Cohort Study." *Diabetes Care* 34, no. 7 (July 2011): 1582–84. https://doi.org/10.2337/dc11-0268.

U.S. Food and Drug Administration. "Advice about Eating Fish: For Women Who Are or Might Become Pregnant, Breastfeeding Mothers, and Young Children." Updated July 2, 2019. https://www.fda.gov/food/consumers/advice-about-eating-fish.

U.S. Food and Drug Administration Center for Food Safety and Applied Nutrition. "Questions and Answers on the Nutrition and Supplement Facts Labels Related to the Compliance Date, Added Sugars, and Declaration of Quantitative Amounts of Vitamins and Minerals: Guidance for Industry (Draft Guidance)." U.S. Department of Health and Human Services, 2017. https://www.fda.gov/media/102614/download.

Index

Acknowledgments

This book has been a product of creativity, hard work, research, and incredible teamwork.

Thank you to the Callisto Media team, for working with Traci and me every step of the way to get this book from idea to fruition. Your patience, dedication, and passion for making this book exactly what the public needs was not unnoticed!

Thank you to Traci, who worked so hard in the kitchen creating balanced and delicious meals that readers are sure to love, and for her patience with me as we worked out every last detail of each recipe to make sure they were simple, delicious, and nourishing for the lovely mamas. You are a rock star!

Thank you to my mentor, Lori Zanini, RD, CDE, who introduced me to the world of cookbook writing and publishing, and who has provided endless support and belief in me over the past many years.

Lastly, thank you to my husband, Kevin, who gave me the push I needed to get this book going and was rooting for me every step of the way. I love you.   –*Joanna*

This was a demanding project that required a lot of people to make it possible!
My children, who simultaneously drain my energy and give me so much life, carried me through this project. Seeing them grow daily has been the best thing in life and I'm so grateful to be their mom.

A special thanks to my mother who was my driving inspiration to learn how to cook. I love how we share a love of food and good food finds. Her support, and God's grace, were instrumental during this time and I'm eternally grateful for the mother and grandmother she is to me and my children.

Thank you to Auntie Jackie for her support, love and encouragement. Her words and cheerfulness are deeply appreciated and I'm thankful to know her better.

Thanks to Joanna whose support, encouragement and compassion during this time has strengthened me. Her beautiful soul has been a bright light to remind me of God's goodness and I'm eternally grateful.

Thank you to the entire Callisto team for creating this book and seeing this through. It will help so many mothers and babies!   –*Traci*

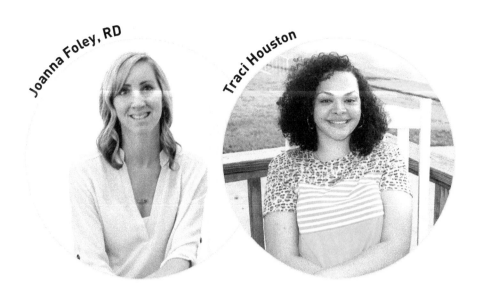

Joanna Foley, RD

Traci Houston

About the Authors

JOANNA FOLEY, RD, has been practicing as a Registered Dietitian for over five years. She has a passion for teaching others how to truly use food as medicine and the best healing tool for their bodies. She is the owner of a virtual nutrition consulting practice, Joanna Foley Nutrition (www.joannafoleynutrition.com), where she strives to help others create the healthiest versions of themselves. In her free time, Joanna enjoys hiking, traveling internationally, cooking new recipes, playing with her pug, and spending time in the sunshine of her city of San Diego, California.

TRACI HOUSTON left a 10-year career in the Air Force to pursue a passion and enrolled in culinary school. While in school, she became pregnant for the first time and got diagnosed with GDM. A subpar experience with her health care team led her to begin blogging recipes for women with GDM. Traci's blog, www.thegestationaldiabetic.com, serves as a recipe blog and resource center addressing common questions and pain points of GDM mothers.

CPSIA information can be obtained
at www.ICGtesting.com
Printed in the USA
BVHW091714270919
559636BV00005B/6